RAPIDLY REVERSIBLE
LOW BACK PAIN

PHYSICAL THERAPY
IN MOTION

505 E. Michigan Ave.
Saline, MI 48176
Tel (734) 944-1005
Fax (734) 944-1303

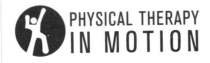

David Oliver, PT, Dip. MDT
Director

Diploma in Mechanical Diagnosis & Therapy
Through The McKenzie Institute International

505 E. Michigan Ave.
Saline, MI 48176

Tel (734) 944-1005
Fax (734) 944-1303

Rapidly Reversible Low Back Pain

An Evidence-Based Pathway
to Widespread Recoveries and Savings

By

Ronald Donelson, MD, MS

SelfCare First, LLC
Hanover, New Hampshire

Ronald Donelson, MD, MS, DipMDT is a board-certified orthopedic surgeon who specialized in non-operative spine care for 20 years, first in private practice and then in academia at The Institute for Spine Care at the State University of New York in Syracuse. He was granted the Diploma in Mechanical Diagnosis & Therapy in 1991 and completed a Master of Science program in 1998 at the Dartmouth Medical School Center for Evaluative Clinical Sciences in New Hampshire. He is currently President of SelfCare First, a consulting, publishing, and low back pain disease management company.

His numerous research publications have focused on the assessment, classification, and non-operative treatment of neck and low back pain. He has also written many chapters, review articles, scientific abstracts and posters and has presented more than one hundred research papers, conference workshops, courses, and symposia in more than 15 countries. *Rapidly Reversible Low Back Pain* is his first book.

Dr. Donelson is an Advisory Editor with the journal *Spine*, an active member of the International Society for the Study of the Lumbar Spine, the North American Spine Society, has been active with the International Forum for Primary Care Research in Low Back Pain, and is currently the Vice President of the American Back Society.

He is married to Lois, his wife of 38 years who, as a physical therapist, also specializes in spine care. They have three married children and three grandchildren.

Figure 14-1 reprinted with the permission of The Free Press, a division of Simon & Schuster Adult Publishing Group, from *Diffusion of Innovations*, Fourth Edition by Everett M. Rogers. Copyright © 1962, 1971, 1983 by The Free Press. All rights reserved.

SelfCare First, LLC, Hanover, New Hampshire

ISBN 978-0-9790387-0-9 (trade paper)

To Lois: my love, my best friend and my partner.

And to my Creator, from whom
comes grace, faith, peace, hope, and love.

Contents

Acknowledgements

In writing this text, I have greatly benefited from the cumulative input of so many colleagues over so many years. This includes spine clinicians of all disciplines, researchers, health policy makers, as well as individuals within the payer community. The aggregate of their perspectives on low back pain, its management, and its scientific investigation have shaped my thinking in a way that, for some reason, is proving to be of such interest to so many that I now pass it on to you in this book in the hope that it will be worthy of your time to read.

I would like to also thank Bruce Fredrickson, Hansen Yuan, and Tom Masten, my spine care colleagues at the Institute for Spine Care in Syracuse, NY, for the opportunity to work with and beside them for many years, and for their enduring support and friendship.

To the many that generously and patiently taught and shared with me over so many years the non-operative management of those struggling with low back pain, I am very grateful.

For those who have now taken their valuable time to review this text, providing so many helpful comments and criticisms that brought much needed assistance to my meager writing skills, I thank you all.

I must further acknowledge six special members of that reviewer group who also contributed to this book's Foreword. Thank you David Ferris, Don Kollisch, Robin McKenzie, Don Murphy, Kevin Spratt, and Todd Wetzel.

You will see that two of these individuals have also played particularly important roles, one in my approach to, and understanding of, low back pain management and the other in molding my view of clinical research strategy. I am forever grateful to Robin McKenzie and Kevin Spratt for all they have taught me.

Finally, I must acknowledge and thank Charles King for his excellence in editing and formatting this text and for his sound guidance throughout the entire publishing process.

Preface

I could have written much of this book fifteen years ago. Along with many other clinicians with experiences similar to mine, I was impressed with many of my low back pain patients' rapid recoveries. But it was and remained disheartening for many years that there was no or so little scientific evidence to document our experience. Consequently, for these many years, I could only have written a descriptive, anecdotal book, whose value would not have justified the effort. Any such writing would need to wait for the scientific evidence to be generated, something I was confident would come in time.

Well, that was then, and this is now. Over these past fifteen years, that evidence has appeared and continues to grow to where it is now sufficiently strong and abundant to warrant me writing and, hopefully, you reading this book.

But you might legitimately ask: if that evidence exists and is published, then why is this book necessary? Aren't there other, even better, sources to read about this type of care and its evidence?

Actually, yes. The evidence is published in prominent spine-related journals. The problem is it is not being acknowledged or sufficiently discussed, because it is not being understood. And that's another big part of the story that needs to be told. There's a much bigger story that requires the linkage of a number of pieces in the hope of providing you with a coherent understanding of how and why it is now finally possible to sort out and successfully treat and prevent large portions of the low back pain challenge.

My goal is to write a scientifically credible presentation of a clinical process that is turning out to be an "evidence-based" pathway to widespread recoveries and cost savings for many people, perhaps the majority of people, suffering from low back pain. But such a process is much different than most of you might think, or what has been portrayed in low back pain clinical guidelines, as you'll discover as you read.

Winston Churchill once said: "A mind is like a parachute, it only functions when it is open." I am hopeful your mind will be open as you read and that perhaps I can help some skeptics to allow the mounting evidence to persuade them to consider these data with fresh eyes. Sir Isaac Newton said: "The human brain can be trained if it belongs to a student who wants to learn." Your reason for reading *Rapidly Reversible* is no doubt to learn. Whether you are a person suffering from low back pain, involved with someone suffering from low back pain, a clinician, a researcher, a payer, or an educator, I feel safe in saying that your personal experience and reality with low back pain thus far is unlikely to represent the whole truth, just as mine is not. Hopefully this book can help us all find more of that whole truth.

The true reward in life is being able to make a difference in people's lives. One of my personal rewards will be to successfully pass on some additional and important portions of the whole truth about low back pain.

Enjoy!

If a writer is so cautious that he never writes anything that can be criticized, he will never write anything that can be read.
If you want to help other people, you have got to make up your mind to write things that some men will condemn.

—Thomas Merton: *Seeds of Contemplation*

Foreword

Comments by Donald Kollisch, F. Todd Wetzel, Kevin F. Spratt, Donald R. Murphy, Robin McKenzie and David M. Ferriss

It will be a very bright day indeed when we have a viable non-operative treatment for Low Back Pain (LBP) due to Degenerative Disc Disease (DDD). That day is closer than we realize, as Dr. Donelson notes in *Rapidly Reversible Low Back Pain*. As supported by an increasing body of reputable scientific knowledge, it is now possible to classify non-specific LBP as well as sciatica into validated subgroups for which there are subgroup specific treatments.

When asked by my long time friend and colleague, Dr. Donelson, to review his manuscript, I had a very pleasant surprise. Far from being a dry summary of scientific data, I found that I literally could not put this book down. This text is a lively and masterful summary of the *misuse* of research methodologies that has led us to miss the point as we continue to ask the wrong research questions, being seduced more by trial design than the actual relevance of trial content. Not only does Dr. Donelson offer penetrating insight into the value of our past and current non-Randomized Controlled Trials (RCTs) and RCT research inventory, but he also proposes truly elegant directions for future research.

This book is also important because of the practical clinical insight into the management of LBP it provides. Arguably, the most important task of the surgeon is patient selection, namely offering the right procedure for the right patient leading to a successful outcome. Not only does MDT have value as a *treatment* technique for LBP due to DDD, it has the additional advantage of helping the surgeon *determine* who would benefit from surgery if MDT is not effective.

For example, many patients thought to be exclusively surgical candidates are still capable of non-surgical recovery if given the opportunity to be assessed using MDT methods delivered by a qualified practitioner. Several published studies document this. One always finds it comforting when the emerging evidence reflects one's own experience: in my nearly twenty years of surgical practice, MDT assessment consistently yields not only clinical success, i.e. good non-surgical outcomes but, as noted above, enhances the precision of my surgical selection process and thereby improves surgical outcomes.

One final point. As one reads the scientific literature, the following should be kept in mind: since MDT assessment and care has not been commonly offered to date in the various surgical studies, one must wonder how many patients would have improved with MDT to where they chose to forgo surgery entirely?

Read and enjoy.

F. Todd Wetzel, MD
Professor of Orthopaedic Surgery and Neurosurgery
Temple University School of Medicine
Philadelphia, PA

As family practitioners, we've all had experience treating our patients with low back pain. We follow the guidelines taught to us by our residency teachers; we follow the formal clinical guidelines published by various groups; or we simply (and reasonably) base our management on our training, reading, and experience. Sadly, not only are our management proposals sometimes hard to sell to our patients, but they so often simply do not work. Yes, our patients sometimes recover—whether due to our medications and PT referrals or simply due to time—but often they don't. And also often, their pain recurs in the future. We also are wary of the downward spiral that we trigger when we use opioid medications.

Most of us want to provide care that doesn't treat the low back as a "black box." We'd rather utilize active interventions rather than passive waiting. And we'd like to have an explanatory model which has educational validity for our patients, is intellectually stimulating, and points to care that works. We need to find alternatives that help patients manage their own low back pain.

Rapidly Reversible Low Back Pain provides the office-based family practitioner or internist with the means to more actively diagnose and treat low back pain. This book's review of the evidence for the causes and treatment of back pain is comprehensive and compelling and its recommendations for future research are interesting for the academic.

While some of us may find such a thorough review of research to be more than we care to wade through, it nevertheless nicely explains why the methods it advocates are not more prominently featured in low back pain clinical guidelines.

So I would encourage perseverance through these sections, because the rest of the book provides a refreshing, evidence-based approach to objectively determine non-pharmacologic means of helping our patients gain control of their pain and recover more quickly and simply. The recommended care promotes objective decision-making and offers new insights into avoiding the need for medication, imaging, or specialist referral, including for low back surgery.

Donald Kollisch, MD
Department of Community and Family Medicine
Dartmouth-Hitchcock Medical Center
Lebanon, NH

My training is as a psychometrician, research methodologist, and statistician. Early in my training, I learned a practical lesson from a speaker about levels of evidence. The lessons learned were that, generally speaking, the lowest form of evidence is when an advocate finds that their approach is better, and the highest form of evidence is when an advocate finds that a competing approach is better.

Since Dr. Donelson is an unabashed advocate for the McKenzie/ Mechanical Diagnosis & Therapy (MDT) paradigm, for the casual reader, and certainly for those "competing" with the MDT approach, this book might be classified as an example of the lowest form of evidence. I would argue otherwise for a number of reasons. First, Dr. Donelson does not attempt to camouflage his position in the hope of convincing those more likely to believe evidence reported by a neutral observer. There is no need to "beware of wolves in sheep's clothing" here. Second, a major theme in the book is about how information becomes "common knowledge" or part of guidelines, rather than the content of that common knowledge. All good scientists must be ever vigilant that "desired" evidence is not touted more than accurate evidence. Third, Dr. Donelson is, in my experience, an unusual advocate who can and will change his mind based on evidence. Fourth, Dr. Donelson has been careful to limit his advocacy to a clearly defined group of patients, and does not claim to have the answer for every patient presenting with LBP. This is not a "one size fits all" approach.

Finally, and perhaps most importantly, the underlying model for MDT represents a logical and methodologically consistent approach for establishing evidence that is robust in diminishing rival hypotheses for explaining observed outcomes. As carefully and repeatedly reported in the book, the MDT system, and much of the research done to evaluate it, has focused on firmly linking assessment with diagnosis, followed by providing theoretical underpinnings for treatment based on the diagnosis, and then carefully evaluating patient outcomes to inform treatment modifications. As a reasonably neutral outside observer, the series of studies conceived and implemented to evaluate MDT, so well-documented by Dr. Donelson, is impressive.

However, given the current state of so-called "evidence-based" low back care, it seems safe to say that the medical community as a whole sends too many patients down the more costly, invasive, and not necessarily more efficacious surgical path than the far less costly, non-invasive, and usually more efficacious MDT path. This is understandable in the case of the surgeons, and maybe even for general practitioners who might feel safer in sending patients down the more traveled path, but for payers to be willing to spend so much more for care, with no strong evidence that patients will benefit more, is hard to understand.

If the existing MDT-based research is accurate, with 70% of acute and 50% of chronic idiopathic LBP cases, as well as sciatica, successfully treated with subgroup-specific interventions, it seems to me this would allow the clinical and scientific community a fabulous opportunity to more closely focus on finding new or existing treatments efficacious for the remaining 30 and 50 percent of LBP patients. This would represent a major paradigm shift in treating patients with LBP, similar to what was observed in Dentistry in the 1950s and 60s in the United States, where virtual eradication of tooth decay due to broadly adopted preventative measures allowed the profession to move away from filling cavities and focus on other aspects of oral disease and care.

Kevin F. Spratt, Ph.D.
Department of Orthopaedic Surgery
Dartmouth Medical School
Lebanon, NH

The much-vaunted randomized controlled trial has been severely limited in its role in providing useful information and solutions for the LBP epidemic. In *Rapidly Reversible Low Back Pain*, Dr. Donelson offers a research strategy for effectively dealing with these deficiencies that brings evidence-based common sense to this epidemic problem. He does this first by exposing the short-sightedness of the health care system's past and present response, and then offers solutions, backing his recommendations with solid evidence.

Much of the confusion regarding LBP arises from the fact that it so often becomes a multifactorial problem. Psychosocial factors, deconditioning, and central pain hypersensitivity likely all play a role in perpetuating chronic LBP. In *Rapidly Reversible Low Back Pain,* Dr. Donelson brings badly needed logic, common sense, *and evidence* to this complex problem and, for the first time, places psychosocial factors in their proper perspective.

In my experience, there is no more powerful way to remedy a patient's fear and psychological distress than to do as Dr. Donelson emphasizes: provide each patient with specific maneuvers that first reduce his or her own pain and then either keep it away or enable him or her to deal effectively with it should it recur. He also doesn't minimize the importance of psychosocial and other factors but puts it all in proper context, providing a practical approach to dealing effectively with the problem as a whole.

As a practitioner whose training focused on manual treatments, I found the chapter on manual therapy particularly interesting. It contained important messages for all manual practitioners, including this essential message: manual therapy can be a very useful tool if used for the right purposes, but it can also cause great harm—not from actual tissue injury but from something far more damaging in the long run—patient dependency.

Rapidly Reversible Low Back Pain is a must-read for anyone interested in having a major impact on the LBP epidemic.

Donald R. Murphy, DC, DACAN
Clinical Director, Rhode Island Spine Center
Clinical Assistant Professor, Brown University Medical School
Adjunct Associate Professor of Research, New York Chiropractic College
Providence, RI USA

Of course from my own point of view, it is a very important book that Dr Donelson has presented here. It is the most comprehensive review yet of my work.

I am likewise pleased that the content so precisely draws attention to the flaws in the scientific process which are exposed so accurately here. It is deplorable that those responsible for issuing guidelines for the management of people with common mechanical back pain have seen fit to spurn a system of treatment that fulfils and provides in so many ways all of the requirements that they have said are essential if we are to improve patient care of the back. Classification, reliability, validity, safety, self care, patient independence and efficacy have all been demonstrated in the many studies presented in this book.

When will they ever learn?

Robin McKenzie, CNZM, OBE. FCSP. (Hon) FNZSP. (Hon) Dip MT.
Raumati Beach.
New Zealand

Dr. Donelson has made an outstanding contribution to our understanding of the assessment and management of low back pain by laying out clearly and concisely the extensive evidence supporting the incorporation of the Mechanical Diagnosis and Therapy paradigm for the assessment and management of low back pain. He constructively presents simple and logical research remedies to advance more rapidly our understanding of LBP and to identify more effective assessment and management methods than what have been produced over the past 25 years.

This book should be of great value to clinicians, researchers, managed care and disease management organizations, and the patients they serve.

David M. Ferriss, MD, MPH, Medical Officer
Clinical Program Development
CIGNA HealthCare

Introduction

*My books are water. Those of great geniuses are wine.
Fortunately, everybody drinks water.*

—Mark Twain

Don't skip this!

Rapidly Reversible Low Back Pain is a story. As such, it is important
to read it from beginning to end, starting here with the Introduction.
Though you may decide to skim some sections that present more detail
than you care to tackle, please read it in the order in which it is written
rather than jumping around in search of quick answers to your specific
questions about low back care. This is not a reference book on low back
pain (LBP). The content is presented in this order because each section
builds on prior ones.

Unlike most other books on LBP, this doesn't just re-state the high
prevalence, high cost, yet favorable natural history of acute LBP, and
then cover the conventional clinical guideline recommendations. My
intent is twofold: to enlighten you about controversies and obstacles to
progress within the world of LBP, as well as some very important LBP
clinical characteristics that have immensely important consequences on
how we manage patients with LBP and spend our financial resources.
The attention of most LBP stakeholders (researchers, clinicians, LBP
guideline experts, policy makers, payers, and of course patients) is, and
has been, directed toward their own LBP niches and not always having
sufficient awareness of the big picture.

LBP is a very common and mystifying health challenge. However,
stakeholders in general do not realize that most LBP also happens to
be *reversible* and, very often, *rapidly* so. Although "reversibility" is not
a familiar descriptive term to most of you in the context of LBP, the
phenomenon to which I am referring is not a new discovery at all and,
indeed, is quite familiar to a small sector of LBP clinicians and patients
alike. *Rapidly reversible* is a characteristic of most LBP that needs much
wider exposure, appreciation, and understanding across the entire
spectrum of LBP players.

There is also considerable evidence now that validates this reversibility and that evidence is largely what has motivated me to write this book. This single LBP characteristic has the potential, if more broadly understood and utilized, to greatly improve the quality of care while dramatically reducing its cost.

What is so impressive about *rapidly reversible LBP* is that this extraordinary phenomenon helps solve most individuals' LBP. And how many of those would otherwise be still struggling with their pain and disability, or their many recurrences?

A solution for most LBP? Is that possible? Is there something even better than the natural history or the recommendations of LBP clinical guidelines? Is there something that can prevent pain from returning? Read on. When you have finished this book, you will be enlightened about *rapid reversibility* and may even be motivated to seek out more information.

Before I review this evidence later in the book, I will tell you about another important and disturbing piece of this story: the extent to which so many LBP stakeholders have been overlooking this *rapid reversibility* and all its supportive research. There's truly been an evidence-based elephant in the room, recognition of which can no longer be avoided or ignored by the so-called LBP experts. Why is something so effective, with so much scientific evidence, and in such widespread use worldwide, disregarded by many experts?

I'll be relating the quiet transition underway in how we care for LBP. But considering the strength of the published supportive evidence, it is remarkable how slow this transition has been. Consequently, the unnecessary consumption of vast sums of money persists while millions worldwide suffer unnecessarily. This book is intended to accelerate our progress in those two important areas.

In writing *Rapidly Reversible Low Back Pain*, I want my readers to learn, to understand, and to "get it." In describing and discussing these concepts, you may find me repetitive. I make no apologies for that, since repetition is often so important to learning and understanding.

What type of LBP stakeholder are you?

While you may have come across this book on your own, more likely someone has given it to you to read because they feel there are important things here that you should know as a member of one of the five stakeholder groups.

You may be a member of one of the two specific groups who suffer directly from LBP. The first group is the obvious one: those individuals who personally experience pain in their lower backs, and those individuals' families. There are a lot of you out there. You seek care but are commonly given unproven, questionably effective treatments. Desperate, many of you turn to "alternative care" methods, some of which have, as yet, meager scientific basis. Failure to improve too often brings referral for spinal imaging, injections and even surgery. While I have not written this book specifically to those of you with LBP, it is certainly written about you, and written for your benefit. The means to better address your suffering is my primary motivation in writing this book.

There is a second group of readers who are also suffering from LBP, but in a different way. You are the payers, especially employers, whether small or large self-insured companies. Your suffering is economic rather than physical pain. You watch and tremble as your employees and their dependants with LBP go off to consult with a wide assortment of clinicians in your community who prescribe an equally wide array of treatments. Some of your employees recover quickly, but many do so very slowly or just partially, and some not at all. Most of you employers and health and safety personnel see some treatments work better than others, most of them unsupported in LBP guidelines, and some that may stretch your sense of appropriateness.

Two other stakeholders who are prominent players and whose work is discussed at length throughout the book are the LBP clinicians and researchers. These groups differ from patients and payers in that neither are personally confronted to any great degree with either form of pain (physical or economic) felt by patients and payers. Indeed, some clinicians are reaping substantial economic rewards as they try to address non-resolving LBP. Some skeptics have suggested that there are some clinicians, researchers, guideline experts, and LBP policymakers who are not open to hearing about LBP solutions, convinced that no widely effective treatment exists and, therefore by extension, that the treatments they offer are as good as any. Sometimes treatments even seem to benefit the treating clinicians more than they do their patients.

The final stakeholder group in whom I have a special interest is those involved in the disease management industry. Disease management programs target most chronic diseases, focusing especially on self-care strategies that influence the prevention of disease complications. Disease management programs targeting LBP have not as yet flourished, largely because of the weak and non-specific guideline recommendations which are insufficient for building a robust, cost-saving disease management program. Key ingredients for a successful disease management program for LBP are contained in this book.

Many clinicians and researchers who read *Rapidly Reversible Low Back Pain* will be challenged. Others might dismiss it as just another self-serving effort to promote a paradigm of care that they view as having only meager evidence to support its use. However, some of the evidence I'll present will challenge some of the sacred clinical and research models that have been espoused, taught, written about, and advocated by some of these same LBP experts. I am hopeful that reading *Rapidly Reversible Low Back Pain* will open some minds to re-evaluate these long-standing models and paradigms, some of which have failed to demonstrate sufficient efficacy to remain recommended. By focusing primarily on published research and scientific evidence, my intent is to help readers grasp the validity of the message I'm bringing. I've also tried to acknowledge when I am drawing on my own and others' experience in the absence of substantial data.

It is my hope that *Rapidly Reversible Low Back Pain* will be both an eye and mind opener that will be a catalyst of progress in our collective understanding of LBP, bringing much needed alignment of thought and incentives amongst LBP stakeholders.

The economic pain of LBP

The minimal progress over the past 25 years in learning either the cause of most LBP or how to cost-effectively best manage it has resulted in steadily rising direct and indirect costs. Estimates of the annual U.S. price tag have grown well into the tens of billions of dollars, with the highest annual U.S. estimate being over $90 billion.[92] As the business world is struggling with how to manage their growing health care overhead, LBP continues to be their greatest single expense in the huge musculoskeletal domain.

Most health care economists agree that a large percentage of this high cost is unnecessary and that medical care and disability claims are excessive. But how do we begin to control and diminish those costs? Can cost-control decisions be based on objective clinical decision-making after evaluating individual patients, or can it only occur through policy and reimbursement changes based on generalizing RCT results, systematic reviews, and guideline findings? And if we work to decrease the cost of care, will these cost reductions be accompanied by a decrease in the quality of care?

I think not. After you have read *Rapidly Reversible Low Back Pain*, I think you will agree that the quality of care can be improved while the costs are reduced, both dramatically so.

A special message to employers, occupational health and work safety personnel

For employers, occupational health and work safety personnel, this book at first glance may seem like far more reading about LBP than you ever wanted to tackle. On the other hand, with your familiarity with the high variability of low back care in your community, it is my hope that you will find this helpful in addressing your concerns, especially your costs. Indeed, I hope to provide you with, and motivate you to take, some action steps to influence low back care in your local environment.

Just like all other stakeholders, employers need more objective measures to determine what care is appropriate and inappropriate for purchase, rather than having to pay for anything and everything that's prescribed by the treating clinicians. The distasteful cost containment alternatives are to either withhold or ration certain forms of care, usually on the basis of LBP clinical guideline recommendations. Simply withholding some forms of care is a very objectionable strategy for employees and certainly for affected clinicians. Toward the end of the book, I've shared some constructive ways for payers to positively influence both the quality and cost of low back care in your workplace and community.

My background

How have I come to write this book? How did a rural general orthopedic surgeon with a sports medicine interest ever end up as a non-operative, academic-based spine care specialist, researcher, and now author? One spine clinician friend has referred to my transition to non-operative care as that of a "recovering surgeon."

My interest in LBP was initially stimulated in the late '70s after first entering general orthopedic practice in northern Vermont. Greg Silva, a very skilled physical therapist, was the only PT in the community and began treating my LBP patients using what to me at the time were rather unorthodox methods, but with some intriguing results. I began to see some low back problems turn around quite quickly. On one hand, I couldn't help but be fascinated yet I had no sense of the importance of what he was showing and teaching me.

For the next few years, I observed and was increasingly impressed by many more patients' rapid recoveries using these spine care methods that I was never taught during my years of orthopedic training. I soon learned that hardly any other orthopedic surgeons were familiar with these methods either.

It became clear over time that these treatment techniques needed some research and documentation, but I had no idea or training in how to do that. I became interested in relating and teaching other clinicians about this, all of which led to my joining the Orthopedic Department at the State University of New York in Syracuse in 1988 where a group of us spine specialists formed the Institute for Spine Care to facilitate the delivery of our tertiary spine care. By that time, I had also become involved with several research spine societies where I further learned that most spine physicians were not only unfamiliar with, but were quite apathetic toward learning anything about these methods that were to me so impressive.

Over the past 15–20 years, many have published research and review articles supportive of this form of clinical assessment and decision-making. And, although I've made well over one hundred presentations at clinical and research conferences over the past 20 years, I have never received such positive, enthusiastic feedback as when I recently began to deliver shorter versions of the big picture I'm attempting to present in this book.

There are essentially three converging factors that have compelled me to write this book. First is my extensive personal clinical experience, not unlike many other clinicians now, identifying and then helping people correct their own *rapidly reversible LBP*. Second, the ever-loudening call from leading LBP experts for fundamental changes in how LBP is being researched and clinically managed. Third, and perhaps most importantly, the emergence over the past fifteen years of a body of scientific evidence specifically supporting the validity of this clinical paradigm.

Overall, only a small percentage of LBP clinicians and researchers understand this paradigm well. For the rest, this clinical pathway to recoveries and cost-savings has unfortunately remained either unknown or certainly greatly misunderstood for too long. It is hoped that this book will assist in remedying this situation by providing a better understanding of LBP for the purpose of improving outcomes and dramatically dropping the huge LBP overhead.

How this book is organized

In order to fully appreciate where we are, there is value in looking at the past twenty years of clinical LBP management and research efforts to get a sense of the fundamental issues impeding our progress despite so many people's hard work. Part 1 also examines current theories and knowledge of the many LBP disciplines contributing to the high varia-tion in care that then drives the cost of care higher and higher. Please don't skip over these early chapters. Understanding them is critical in providing the context necessary to see the big picture that represents both the forest and the trees.

Part 2 turns to LBP research, examining and pondering its lack of productivity in discovering the causes of, and solutions to, LBP. I also describe and illustrate a simple, yet highly effective and badly needed research rationale and strategy that a growing number think needs widespread consideration and adoption to more quickly advance our discovery of LBP understanding.

Part 3 introduces the phenomenon of *rapidly reversible LBP* and its related management paradigm. I review the extensive, yet largely over-looked, evidence documenting the successful treatment and recovery of the majority of LBP sufferers using individualized self-care methods rather than one-size-fits-all, "silver bullet" care recommended in cur-rent clinical guidelines.

Parts 4 and 5 discuss important implications and benefits of iden-tifying LBP subgroups and implementing this paradigm on a broad scale. The published evidence speaks clearly of the many expensive and completely unnecessary diagnostic and therapeutic interventions that are commonly utilized today as a result of today's current diverse care of LBP. This problem is directly related to the widespread lack of familiarity with *rapidly reversible LBP.*

Part 6 then offers ways to bring this form of care to more patients so they too can rapidly reverse their LBP and their payers can save large sums of money by helping more of their employees and members avoid prolonged care and high cost interventions.

The bottom line: *Rapidly Reversible Low Back Pain* is an important read for payers.

To get started, let's consider these questions. . . .

- If acute low back pain is as self-limiting (recovers on its own) as most experts and clinical guidelines say it is, why are we spending so much money on it?
- Given that LBP guidelines recommend the same treatment for 85% of sufferers, do all those people suffer from the same type of LBP? If so, then why are there so many different treatments utilized for the same problem? If not, then how can we tell one type from another in order to determine the best treatment for each type?
- Is there a way to tell at the outset of care whether an individual with LBP will, or can, recover or not? Are there ways to significantly speed that recovery or even help some recover that wouldn't otherwise do so?
- How can we improve our management of LBP without increasing the cost of care? Is it a requirement to pay more in order to improve our outcomes?
- How often do people with LBP *unnecessarily* undergo expensive diagnostic or treatment interventions? Is there a way to determine if, when, or how often that happens?
- And finally, with over 1,000 randomized controlled trials of back pain and disability, and dozens of systematic reviews and guidelines, why are we not finding explanations for LBP's prominence, its causes, and its best treatments?

It is my position that we do not have to wait another 15–20 years to find answers to these questions. I believe some very important and constructive answers are available now. I intend to provide those answers and the evidence to support them within the pages of *Rapidly Reversible Low Back Pain*. By familiarizing ourselves with the existing evidence, much of which has been ignored in most guidelines, we are enabled to take the necessary steps to implement badly needed changes. We can begin to implement these changes now, today, not ten or twenty years from now.

Hang on to your hats. We're heading off on a bit of an adventure. If quality patient care is your priority, and you also wish to decrease your cost of low back care, then you should find this book instructive.

PART 1
The Low Back Pain Dilemma

Chapter 1
A Symptom, Not a Diagnosis!

Clinical guidelines are primarily created out of concern for the high variability and associated high cost of care. This variability in care is typically related to a large degree to the arbitrariness in selecting treatments, suggesting the need for a better understanding of the clinical problem being treated.

The elusiveness of quality care throughout medicine has been especially noted by David Eddy, MD, PhD, and Senior Advisor for Health Policy and Management at Kaiser Permanente in California. In his book entitled "Clinical Decision Making: From Theory to Practice" he states: "The plain fact is that many decisions made by physicians appear to be arbitrary—highly variable, with no obvious explanation. The very disturbing implication is that this arbitrariness represents, for at least some patients, suboptimal or even harmful care."[57] Indeed, the quality of clinical decision-making is always compromised to the extent that there is a lack of sufficient knowledge or characterization of each patient's condition.

Confronted with the tension of poor quality care driving up costs, clinical guideline panels, in an effort to improve the quality of that care, are mandated to review the pertinent literature, determine the best evidence-based treatments, and then disseminate their recommendations. Clinical guidelines have now been developed in most health care domains. Likewise, warranted by its high costs and variation in care, low back pain (LBP) is no exception. Or is it?

Actually, LBP is quite a notable exception, since fundamentally it is neither a diagnosis nor a disease process. It is, of course, merely a symptom. But why does a symptom warrant clinical guidelines, not to mention even separate guidelines targeting the acute (recent onset) form of the symptom vs. the chronic form?

Consider this perspective. Where are the "Chest Pain" or "Abdominal Pain" guidelines? Or guidelines for elbow or knee pain? So why LBP? Is it because we have a better understanding of the various causes of those other kinds of pain, whereas there remains great uncertainty as to the cause of the vast majority of LBP?

If an individual with LBP sought care from ten clinicians representing different specialties or disciplines, she could conceivably receive as many as ten different explanations for her pain and receive prescriptions for just as many different treatments.

Alternatively, if you were to ask a group of clinicians how they treated chest pain, and I have done this with audiences during presentations, there is typically only one response, and that response is in the form of a question: "What kind of chest pain?" This response is based on the common recognition of different types of chest pain that demand distinctly different forms of treatment.

So why isn't our response the same regarding how to best treat LBP? "What kind of LBP?" Looking at that question, rather than how best to treat LBP, is the first important step in our journey toward bringing order and understanding to how we prescribe and pay for low back care.

Chapter 2

The Root of the Low Back Pain Dilemma

It has been thirty years since Dr. Alf Nachemson, one of the world's experts on the subject of LBP, authored the lead article in the inaugural issue of the journal *Spine*[24] in which he stated that, in the great majority of patients with low back pain (LBP), no clear diagnosis or explanation for their pain could be found.[106]

Ten years later, the Quebec Task Force (QTF) on Activity-Related Spinal Disorders, the first-ever comprehensive LBP literature review, said a similar thing: "There is so much variability in making a diagnosis that this initial step routinely introduces inaccuracies which are then further confounded with each succeeding step in care." The resulting diagnosis "is the fundamental source of error. . . . Faced with uncertainty, physicians become inventive."[132]

While no one, to my knowledge, has ever challenged that position regarding our fundamental source of error, to what extent has it been addressed?

In the eighteen years since that QTF report, many LBP clinical guidelines have been published. If we search them for the "best evidence" for how to make a *diagnosis or classify* LBP, what is immediately apparent is the brevity with which the topic has typically been addressed, especially when compared with the exhaustive discourses regarding LBP treatment. Historically, the major focus of all guidelines has been on randomized controlled trials (RCTs) designed to compare the effects of two or more LBP *treatments*. The meager information presented regarding *diagnosing* the causes of LBP is of little help in addressing these fundamental challenges raised by Nachemson and the QTF.

Again, David Eddy agrees with the QTF's views.[57] Two years prior to the 1987 QTF report, he provided a bibliography that listed more than 400 articles addressing the essential need of beginning with an accurate diagnosis. "A correct decision about an intervention requires that a patient's condition be diagnosed correctly. Substantial variations in what physicians see have been reported in virtually every aspect of the diagnostic process, from taking a history, to doing a physical examination, reading laboratory tests, performing pathological diagnosis, and recommending treatment."

What is an RCT?

For those less familiar with this type of research design, the randomized clinical trial (RCT) attempts to answer this specific question: for a selected group of patients, what are the likely effects of one treatment compared with another? By randomly assigning similar subjects to various treatment interventions, both recognizable and unrecognizable biases in subject selection are controlled across the treatments. It is then conceptually easier to attribute observed differences between the groups' outcomes to the treatments that are being compared. For similar reasons and justification, Cochrane methodologists and various clinical guideline protocols consider little else beyond the RCT design in reaching their treatment conclusions and recommendations.

Now here we are in the 21st century, and LBP remains a diagnostic enigma. Winston Churchill, when attempting to forecast Russia's actions, once used this appropriate phrase: "a riddle wrapped in a mystery inside an enigma."[29] The diagnostic challenge of LBP naturally has a profound effect on the quality of our treatment decision-making. As Dr. Gunnar Andersson, a prominent spine surgeon and researcher at Rush Presbyterian St. Luke's Medical Center in Chicago, has stated: "Our treatment success rate can be no better than our diagnostic success rate."[7]

LBP clinical guideline conclusions

The position on LBP assessment and classification held by the most recently published international acute LBP guidelines, the 2004 European Guidelines, is worthy of review.[143] In addressing the topic of how best to classify acute LBP, these guidelines state: "A simple and practical classification, which has gained international acceptance, is by dividing acute low back pain into three categories—the so-called 'diagnostic triage' "(see Figure 2–1). They then go on to describe their three LBP subgroups:

1. Serious spinal pathology: the so-called "red flag" conditions such as tumors, infection, fractures, cauda equina syndrome, or intra-abdominal pathologies that present as LBP.

2. Nerve root / radicular pain: those patients with sciatica and neurological deficits consistent with a herniated intervertebral disc.

3. Non-specific low back pain; i.e., "everyone else." Sometimes referred to as "simple back ache," this group is most often characterized by the absence of any red flag or nerve root forms of LBP.

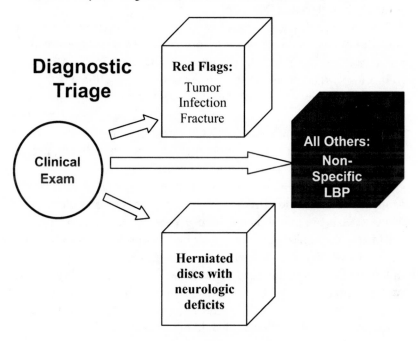

Figure 2–1: The "diagnostic triage."

The "international acceptance" of the diagnostic triage referred to in these guidelines appears to be born out in a published review of eleven international LBP guidelines, all of which acknowledged this same means of classifying or "diagnosing" LBP.[79] What is disconcerting however is that the European Guidelines go on to acknowledge that "there is little scientific evidence on the diagnostic triage (level D)." They then clarify the definition of "Level D evidence," meaning "No evidence; i.e., No diagnostic studies."

So at this most fundamental step in managing LBP, where the QTF states all our problems begin, our most recent guidelines present a means of classification they, on one hand, claim has "gained international acceptance" by most international guidelines, but, on the other, has *little or no scientific evidence.* What are we to conclude? With little or no evidence, such "international acceptance" can only be on the basis of a consensus classification, not only amongst the panel members working on each guideline, but across all these many guidelines. A spine research colleague suggested this resembled what the economist John Kenneth Galbraith described when he coined the term "conventional wisdom," defining it as "the conventional view that serves to protect us from the painful job of thinking."[67]

But, as we shall see, the consensus appears to stop right there with guideline panel members since by no means is there widespread acceptance of the diagnostic triage amongst LBP clinicians.

It is also worth noting that no international guideline has thus far acknowledged any other LBP classification scheme, though they exist, suggesting they are quite comfortable with this evidence-lacking diagnostic triage where the bulk of patients are assigned to the non-specific LBP subgroup, further suggesting that they have no distinguishing characteristics or differing treatment needs.

For the record, at least two classification systems have been prominently investigated and validated over the past fifteen years. But neither their existence nor any of their evidence has ever been acknowledged in any international LBP guideline to my knowledge. So the obvious question arises: why is a classification system with no evidence attracting such widespread acknowledgement while those with considerable evidence are being ignored? We'll explore this further in the next chapter.

For now, let's go with the "international acceptance" of the diagnostic triage, in which case we would do well to modify Figure 2–1 to more accurately reflect the actual prevalence of these three subgroups. Figure 2–2 gives us a much better visual of this classification. What is so ironic, even misleading, about calling this a "diagnostic" classification is that the 85% classified have no identifiable diagnosis! How can we call it a "diagnostic" scheme? Some feel a much more appropriate label for this classification system would be "the black box model" or classification.[14] I agree, and will use this term often.

Of course, there is value in acknowledging the two small categories of LBP where we are able to make a diagnosis. The first where we can often confidently make a diagnosis is the herniated disc or nucleus pulposus. Such a diagnosis is made in the presence of three essential findings: sciatica (a pattern of pain distribution extending to the lower leg or foot), a related neurological deficit (signs of nerve compression from the displaced disc nucleus), and confirmatory advanced imaging demonstrating this herniation. We will discuss this subgroup at some length in Chapter 10.

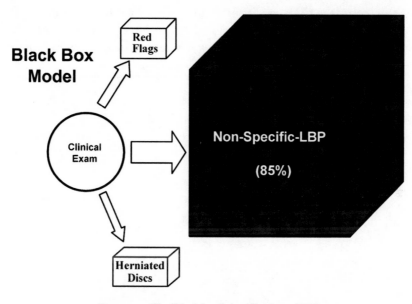

Figure 2–2: The "black box" classification of LBP.

The second small category is the "red flag" subgroup that I will not be spending any significant time addressing. The identification and management of these more serious and urgent pathologies are well-described in many other texts.[103, 151]

More than 25 years have passed since Nachemson made his statement regarding our inability to identify a diagnosis for 85% of LBP patients. Regrettably, according to our more recent guidelines, this non-specific-LBP subgroup remains the only available "diagnostic" home for 85% of LBP. And that's not much of a home if you are the one struggling with LBP and looking for a solution, or the one paying for their care.

In truth, applying the term "non-specific LBP" to 85% of LBP is a meaningless and unproductive label. That point has been emphatically made by Gordon Waddell, an orthopedic surgeon from Scotland and, ironically, a very prominent influence in many international LBP guidelines. He wrote: "the label 'nonspecific back pain' is simply not a useful diagnosis. . . . It is intellectually and scientifically inadequate and fails to provide any biological basis for real understanding." It "betrays our ignorance and leads to failure of communication, and to confusion and lack of confidence."[148]

Now that's a sobering view of the diagnostic label applied to 85% of acute LBP patients by most international acute LBP clinical guidelines. As stated by the QTF, our inability to make a diagnosis for most LBP patients lies at the heart of all our problems, creating immensely important and expensive consequences. There is value in spending some time looking at those consequences.

Chapter 3

Two Consequences of No Low Back Pain Diagnosis

No single factor in the low back pain (LBP) dilemma is more critical than our lack of either a diagnosis or a dependable means of classification for the majority of individuals with LBP. Although there are many consequences to the lack of a diagnosis, I believe two in particular stand out.

The first is the resulting and understandable high variation in low back care that leads to our high cost for low back care. A second, but not so obvious, consequence is clinicians' widespread non-compliance with current LBP clinical guideline recommendations. These two items are curiously intertwined and together expose our fundamental need for progress, on the part of both LBP clinicians and researchers, in classifying LBP patients.

Let's look a little deeper at these two consequences and the perpetual counter-productive cycle they have created.

1. High variation in care: remedies, too-numerous-to-count,

in search of a cure

Perhaps the most obvious consequence of our inability to make a diagnosis for most LBP is the freedom granted to clinicians of all disciplines and specialties to label most LBP patients rather arbitrarily, based on each clinician's proprietary educational background, unproven theories, and often dogmatic views regarding the mechanisms of back pain production.

Recall the Quebec Task Force's (QTF) warning: "There is so much variability in making a diagnosis that this initial step routinely introduces inaccuracies which are then further confounded with each succeeding step in care." The resulting diagnosis "is the fundamental source of error. . . . Faced with uncertainty, physicians become inventive" (Figure 3–1).

But how can there be so many diagnoses and labels for the same symptom and even for the same patient by different clinicians?

Of course, we must first acknowledge the many types of clinicians that care for LBP. Within the medical field alone, there are the primary care groups (family practice, emergency room medicine, internal medicine, even pediatrics) as well as many specialties, like rheumatology, neurology, physiatry, orthopedic surgery, neurosurgery, occupational health, anesthesia, pain medicine, and even psychology. Then there are the osteopaths and chiropractors; i.e., manual medicine doctors. Additionally, the allied health fields are very active, made up of physical therapists, massage therapists, and a host of alternative medicine practitioners with great variation in low back care within each of those fields.

Isn't it ironic and, perhaps, revealing that, after 25 or more years of voluminous, apparently high quality, clinical research, systematic reviews, and guideline recommendations, so many LBP sufferers are now flocking to alternative care methods, where there is such a deficiency in science (see Figure 3–1)?

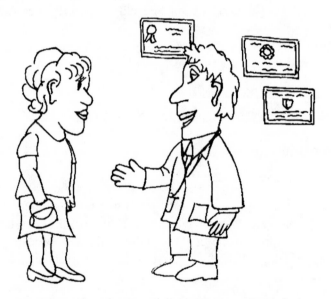

Figure 3–1: "It's a guess, but a highly educated guess."

Of course, most clinicians are very sincere in their desire to provide quality care and strive hard to do so, yet there are so many different ways in which LBP is evaluated and managed.

Many clinical disciplines resemble craft groups that have been trained to use unique methods, taught by their mentors in their respective "craft schools" or residencies' widely disparate LBP concepts and interventions. What is common to one of these groups is a mystery to others. The inaccuracies, variations, and shortcomings that typify so much of this training seem to be captured by this statement (source unknown): "Half of what we learned in medical [insert physical therapy, chiropractic, osteopathic, etc.] school is false. Unfortunately, we don't know which half."

Each clinical discipline teaches its own unproven theories of pain production wrapped in a belief system that includes rationales for justifying and defending its own LBP classification and management method. This training, indeed the culture and language, are passed down mostly unchallenged from one generation to the next, resulting in rigid belief systems.

Noticeably absent in most training programs are faculty members (and consequently their students who emulate them) with a curiosity and skepticism regarding the validity of the assumptions, beliefs and notions that stand as pillars of the discipline. These pillars are to be defended by the faithful, despite the absence of rigorous scientific validation regarding any of the fundamental clinical processes: patient assessment methods, outcome-prediction, pain-generating models, clinical algorithms, diagnostic terminology and, of course, treatments and outcome measurement. Students' educational resources are usually limited to their mentors' content, reasoning, and scope of understanding, and only infrequently, if ever, would they question these esteemed role models. After all, regardless of the discipline in which you seek training, how could anyone who has attained such a prestigious academic position be wrong?

Due to the wide disparities in these clinical approaches, these clinical groups become very exclusive, often driven by economic competition with one another, and related to their unique terminology and diagnostic labeling that seriously compromises, even prevents, effective communication across groups. One's comfort and security within one's own system is an understandable and natural outcome, but these are often closely tied to a closed-mindedness toward anything or anyone that challenges that system and one's comfort zone.

Consequently, the various LBP approaches to evaluating and providing a diagnosis for patients are too often driven more by each discipline's theories of pain production than by anything specifically related to individual patient's clinical presentation. The patient evaluation might then be characterized by the common saying (again, source unknown): "We seek what we look for and find what we know."

This has led to the erection of walls that separate these disciplines, walls that are highly re-enforced by the competition to capture a greater share of the LBP market, which becomes the driving force behind the familiar "turf battles" that evoke various local, state, and national political, legislative, and marketing efforts.

One study very nicely illustrated this wide variation in care by surveying what tests clinicians of various disciplines commonly ordered when evaluating LBP patients.[27] Not surprisingly, neurosurgeons ordered far more spinal imaging studies than did non-surgeons, while neurologists focused on EMGs and rheumatologists on blood tests.

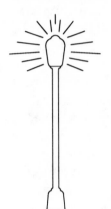

So we learn to look for what we are trained to understand and that with which we are familiar and comfortable. Some have referred to this as the "street light phenomenon"; i.e., looking for the lost item only under the street light, where it would be easiest to see and find.

That all these disciplines uniformly disagree with "the black box model" of LBP classification, where 85% are viewed as having non-specific LBP, is evident when one reviews some revealing survey findings. Despite medical doctors', physical therapists', chiropractors' and osteopaths' widely different approaches to LBP, 93% of 650 surveyed indicated they did not view non-specific LBP as a single condition and instead attempted to classify and treat their patients based on their own system of classification.[74]

What is the validity evidence for these many classification systems? A follow-up study by the same investigators reported that most of these same clinicians routinely gave pathoanatomic diagnostic labels to patients with non-specific LBP, even though there was scant or, at best, controversial evidence for such labels.[73] Yet how is this different than clinical guidelines that recommend we classify patients using their "diagnostic triage" for which there is no supportive evidence?

The role of patients' expectations and satisfaction

Another factor that influences clinicians' diagnoses is their patients' expectations. Patients typically want three things: to get rid of their pain, an explanation for it, and reassurance that it is nothing serious. Wishing to satisfy their patients' expectations, clinicians routinely turn to their leading, even though unproven, theory of pain production and provide their favorite explanation or diagnosis.

It is a rare doctor who is comfortable telling patients "I don't know what's causing your pain," or "you suffer from what we call "non-specific LBP, which means we don't know the cause." Instead, many confidently explain the cause of the patient's LBP, motivated in large part by their desire to please their patients. They rely on theories and pain mechanisms they have been taught in school or at their most recent spine conference. Thus, diagnoses are as variable as the training received. The list of possible diagnoses given patients with LBP is extremely long, many of which, as described by the QTF, are quite "inventive." Chiropractors are perhaps the best trained in providing their specific theories of the cause of LBP and routinely provide these explanations coherently to their patients,[23, 70] even though the scientific evidence to support most of these theories is lacking.

Further, in pursuit of a prompt explanation for their back pain, many patients have been "educated" to expect or even request an MRI soon after symptom onset. Such demands for inappropriate and expensive studies are too often fulfilled by physicians insufficiently educated regarding the limitations of such studies in identifying the cause of the LBP.

Another side of that occurrence was revealed in another survey that showed the extra mile physicians are willing to travel to satisfy their patients' desire to know what is wrong or, more commonly, that nothing is seriously wrong. Physicians acknowledge ordering lumbar MRIs early in their low back care simply as a means of impressing their LBP patients that they are leaving no stone unturned. They do this despite acknowledging their awareness of the low yield from such an intervention. Is it any wonder costs are so high?

Treatment determines diagnosis

Another phenomenon that influences diagnoses is the tendency of some clinicians to select a diagnosis that justifies the use of their favorite, most familiar, comfortable, and perhaps most lucrative, treatment. Naturally, such reverse reasoning provokes the important question of whether a recommended treatment is more beneficial to the patient or the provider, leading to the whimsical phrase: "If all you have is a hammer, everything starts looking like a nail" (Figure 3–2).

Another provocative cartoon shows a surgeon telling his patient: "I just talked to my accountant and it looks like you're going to need surgery." It's often said that it's the little bit of underlying truth that makes things funny.

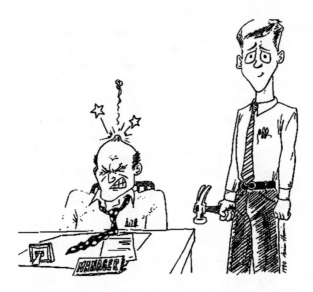

Figure 3-2: If all you have is a hammer, everything starts looking like a nail.

These economic factors were discussed at length in a controversial *New York Times*[24] article in 2003.[1] The article quoted Edward Bentzel, MD, Chairman of the Cleveland Clinic Spine Institute, as estimating "that fewer then half of the spine fusions done today are probably appropriate. He described the current system of paying doctors as "totally perverted." "A lot of technological innovation serves shareholders more than patients," he said. Hardware makers acknowledge giving surgeons millions of dollars in consulting fees, royalty payments and research grants, but say the money promotes technical and medical advances that improve back care.

Does recovery mean your treatment worked?

Despite the many unvalidated diagnostic labels and the equally wide range of related treatments, many with LBP recover. Of course, many individuals with LBP also recover without any treatment. We'll discuss the natural history of LBP shortly but when a clinician prescribes or carries out a treatment and the patient then recovers, both the patient and clinician are quite ready to conclude that the treatment must have been effective. It would also be attractive to conclude that "the diagnosis" must have also been correct. But recovery may well have taken place without any treatment at all or, in some cases perhaps, even more quickly without, or even despite, the selected treatment.

Clinicians can only comfortably prescribe those treatments they are trained and permitted to provide. MDs and osteopathic physicians (DOs), unlike chiropractors and physical therapists, can prescribe medications, but even then, they do so with considerable variability in types, including a range of analgesics, anti-inflammatories, and muscle relaxants, using varying dosages and frequencies.

Even within the physical therapy (P.T.) and chiropractic professions, there is great variability, once again closely tied to their differing training regarding theories of LBP generation and treatment. Prescribing some form of exercise is now very common in both disciplines, yet with considerable variation in intent: some to strengthen muscles, to increase soft-tissue stability, to restore range of movement, for cardiovascular and general fitness purposes, to increase proprioception, to reduce fear of movement as part of a cognitive-behavioral approach, or as part of a return-to-activity program.

P.T.s also commonly utilize other forms of treatment: manual therapy, traction, myofascial and craniosacral care, and a host of other interventions. It is also common to prescribe more than one of these treatments for an individual, often sequentially during different phases of recovery. Such combinations of care are challenging to investigate in a well-controlled RCT.

Chiropractic treatment has been traditionally entrenched in so-called spinal "adjustments" and manipulations, although many are now also prescribing exercise, nutrition modifications, and promoting overall fitness. Many osteopaths now practice as conventional physicians, but many are trained in, and some continue to use, osteopathic manual therapy.

In spite of the diverse treatment modalities across all these disciplines, it seems remarkable that all these approaches, diagnoses and treatments are so commonly used to address the very same patients. The treatment patients receive for their LBP is determined most by the clinician from whom they seek care. Further, it is unfortunate how members of one discipline typically cannot, and even choose not to, communicate effectively with members of other disciplines because, in reality, they are in competition for the LBP dollar, each group striving to muster as much credibility as they can for their respective and usually unproven systems of care. These proprietary systems and terminology prevent meaningful dialogue, which becomes a real source of frustration and irritation to non-clinical stakeholders such as employers, payers, many researchers, and even patients.

Finally, nothing speaks more clearly to the high variation in low back care than spine surgery rates across U.S. geographic areas, as revealed by U.S. Medicare data.[154, 155] Low back surgical rates vary eight-fold from one community or region to the next,[154] with actual differences in patient populations and health care supply explaining only about 10% of this variation.[93] Of particular concern is the recently reported twenty-fold range in rates of lumbar fusions that represents the largest variation seen with any surgical procedure. Medicare spending for fusions increased more than 500% over the past decade and now represents 40% of all Medicare spending on low back care.[154]

As I've said repeatedly, this high variation in care is probably at the root of the high and increasing cost of low back care. Remember that the most recent estimate for the total U.S. annual LBP cost was over $90 billion![92] The problems don't stop there however. In fact, we're just getting started. Let's look at how this wide variation in care drives research and guideline efforts.

Why does high variation in care drive costs so high?

There are no doubt many factors operative here. You can be the judge as to which of these are plausible explanations.

When there is more than one treatment option, both patients and clinicians often mistakenly assume that the more aggressive and more expensive procedure is best. Both groups are often infatuated with the latest advances, the newest technologies, even if such treatments have not been justified by evidence.[22]

Often, the treatments with the highest clinician reimbursement attract more use than they deserve based on the evidence. In a June 2006 *UPI*[24] article, John Wennberg, M.D., the Director of Dartmouth's Center for Evaluative Clinical Sciences and expert in health care efficiency, referred to "supply-driven demand" where care increases simply because care capacity (supply) is high. We spend lots of money developing new technologies that typically drive a big increase in the implementation and then supply of that technology. It's a classic case of *increased supply driving demand*, instead of the other way around. Unlike any other market, health care costs increase simply because expensive interventions are made available, often driven by profit motives, despite inadequate evidence of their efficacy. So we always want the best and most recent technology.

Many doctors also do not take into account patient preferences in treatment and instead recommend the treatments the doctors know and like the best. Many doctors also hold both a financial and a professional interest in treatments they prescribe.

Finally, the public's demands and patient expectations are often directed at immediate and definitive treatment, most of which are expensive, some very expensive. This urgency increases the likelihood of inappropriate treatments, causing their overuse, especially the more expensive ones.

Even low-tech treatments, including some forms of physical and manual therapy, including chiropractic care, can bring excessive costs. With little objective guidance to determine who is and is not a candidate for these treatments, most everyone with LBP receives their clinician's favorite treatment. There is also often no clear end-point for determining when a patient is no longer responding to his or her treatment. Some patients are told they need to continue care to avoid deteriorating again. These forms of passive care are pleasing to many patients who prefer and expect someone else to treat them and assume responsibility for their recovery. Consequently, many people are treated unnecessarily or ineffectively for prolonged periods of time without much if any benefit. The time consumed by this process often adds to the complexity of the problem and finding the ultimate solution.

An interactive cycle involving clinicians, researchers, and guidelines

We know that some form of tension or dissatisfaction with circumstances routinely motivates all us to action, whether in business, in our personal lives, or in health care.

In recent years, this high variation in low back care and the lack of evidence supporting the efficacy of the many types of treatments has led to a cycle of events (Figure 3–3) we have thus far been unable to escape. The right half of this tension-driven cycle depicts the common clinical phenomena I've just described where 85% of LBP patients with no clear diagnosis are given a wide range of diagnostic labels by an equally wide assortment of LBP clinicians of different backgrounds. These many labels then drive the wide range of treatments that, once again, contribute to the high cost of low back care. We might call what is depicted on the right side of this cycle as "high variation care."

One of the important consequences of the tension created by such varied and high cost of care (see "Tension #1" in Fig. 3–3) is the stimulation of research in hopes of finding solutions.

The subsequent research findings then stimulate systematic reviews which then are at the heart of most clinical guidelines, all in hopes of somehow resolving Tension #1, by identifying the best means of either improving the quality of low back care, lowering its cost, or both.

Depicted on the left-side of Figure 3–3 is the huge research effort over the past two decades that has predominately focused on investigating the efficacy of all these many LBP treatments, hoping to identify those most deserving of utilization and reimbursement.

To optimize the chances of identifying truly efficacious treatments, the use of the highest quality in research methodology becomes important. The randomized controlled trial (RCT) is correctly recognized as the highest in the hierarchy of clinical study designs intended to compare the effects of various treatments.

However, with no clear diagnosis for 85% of LBP patients, hundreds of RCTs have had to focus on this large "black box" of patients experiencing non-specific LBP (See Figure 3–4). Not surprisingly, systematic reviews and guideline panels have concluded that these research results are themselves non-specific, and consequently, a "one-size-fits-all" treatment has been recommended.

Consequently, current guidelines attempt to encourage clinicians to accept that most LBP is homogeneous and likely to respond similarly

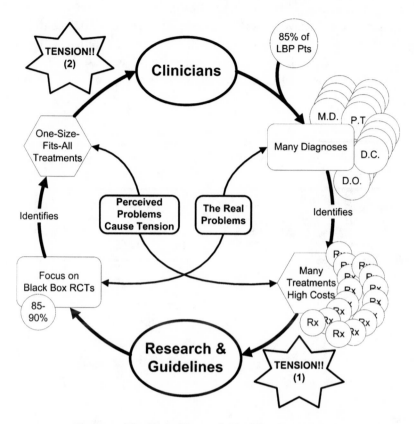

Figure 3–3: The Clinical/Research/Guideline Tension Cycle.

to the same management and treatment. They also recommend that acute LBP care consist of providing advice to patients to remain active, along with reassurance of likely recovery. This care is justified in large part by the perception of a good LBP natural history (see Chapter 4), thereby providing a minimum of formal care. A primary message to those clinicians who treat acute LBP is "don't over-treat."

More extensive treatment may be justified when pain persists for an extended period (at least six weeks), but offering very little treatment initially is the recommended treatment of most guidelines, who feel that is superior to more formal care. Of great concern is that over-treating acute LBP may directly or indirectly teach patients they have something seriously wrong when they perhaps do not.

So the left-side of this Tension Cycle (Figure 3–3) depicts the development and the dissemination of 'non-specific," one-size-fits-all care recommended by most acute LBP guidelines: maintain activity, reassurance of recovery, and avoid bed rest. The essential guideline message is that this form of treatment is what is best for 85% of those with acute LBP. It is this silver bullet, one-size-fits-all recommendation that doesn't sit well with most clinicians and hence introduces a second point of tension.

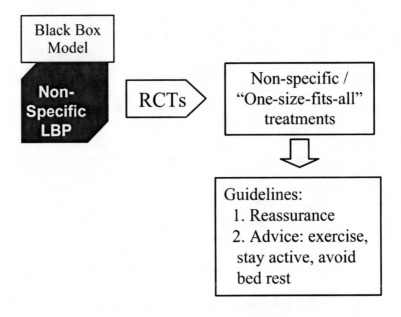

Figure 3–4: Black box RCT outcomes and resulting guideline recommendations.

2. Clinicians' non-compliance with LBP guidelines

Most low back clinicians meanwhile continue to believe in and use their favorite methods to classify their patients into some subgroup to assist them in determining the care they will provide. Most feel that guideline panels fail to appreciate the value of their assessment methods, their favorite and most often used treatment(s), or both. So many clinicians view guideline recommendations as based solely on RCT findings driven by subtle differences in statistical means that are not sufficiently generalizable to their own patients and practices to be of much value. Clinicians' commonly respond: "Researchers and guideline experts aren't working in 'the real world' of patient care like I am." Besides, guideline panelists demonstrate no particular concern about, or provide any strategy to address, the financial viability of those clinical practices that might be inclined to adhere to their recommendations.

In return, guideline panelists, policy makers, and even some payers are asking: "Why are clinicians so non-compliant with guideline recommendations? After all, guidelines are based on a comprehensive review of the best science available today. Clinicians need to be more in tune with what the best research is reporting and what we, as the most knowledgeable of LBP research, have recommended."

Consequently, researchers, guideline advocates and even some payers have concluded that physicians' non-compliance with guideline recommendations is a major part of the problem. But these non-specific, one-size-fits-all treatment guideline recommendations, having evolved from the left side of this cycle, have now created this second important tension point (see "Tension #2" in Figure 3–3) because they directly contradict the views of most clinicians who feel LBP is heterogeneous, with different forms of low back problems best handled with different forms of treatment.

Consistent with this guideline perspective, one prominent international guideline expert stated from the podium at a 2000 international spine conference: "Now that we know how to manage low back pain, the challenge is to get clinicians to implement guideline care." Many would challenge his view that we know how to manage LBP.

Indeed, as you read further, you shall see how little we know about LBP, especially if we were to rely on the conclusions of clinical guidelines only. Yet, holding to the understandable and defendable belief that clinical guideline recommendations represent the best care available, many health policy makers and payers find themselves shifting their focus to how best to bring clinicians into compliance.

A closer look at the Tension Cycle

The left side of this Tension Cycle representing the persistent and rigid focus of the research and guideline community on black box RCTs is no less an obstacle to progress than is clinicians' continued use of unreliable assessments, unvalidated classification systems, unproven pain-generating theories and treatments depicted on the right side of the cycle (see Figure 3–3).

Though rarely if ever acknowledged or discussed, it should not be at all surprising that researchers, systematic reviewers, and guideline panelists are men and women vulnerable to the same foibles as clinicians. They also see only what they are trained and prepared to see. They fall prey to the same characteristic we noted in clinicians: they "see what they look for and find what they know." Thus individual players on either side of this cycle no doubt see through their own lenses the things that they want, or feel they need, to see.

In the center of this Tension Cycle in Figure 3–3, I've labeled the two points in the cycle so often "perceived" to be the problems, and routinely blamed for being such; i.e. too many treatments and high cost on the clinical (right) side and the one-size-fits all treatments derived on the research/guideline (left) side of the cycle. It is important to realize however that "the real problems," also labeled in Figure 3–3, lie rather with our inability to either reliably make a diagnosis or identify and validate LBP subgroups. This single shortcoming is the source of both our high variation in making a diagnosis on the right of the cycle and our unproductive black box RCTs on the left.

Yet, how can we resolve these two tensions when we don't know the causes of LBP? We certainly don't have any tests that identify or reliably confirm the various causes.

Or do we? As we continue, I will introduce you to the abundance of peer-review and generally overlooked research that provides some simple yet substantial answers to these two tensions driving this unproductive cycle in which we're currently stuck. But before going there, we need to re-examine the natural history of LBP since that has such a strong influence on how we view and manage acute LBP. This next chapter will provide the evidence regarding the natural history for acute LBP, and it may not be as optimistic as we have been led to believe by most clinical guidelines and expert consensus.

Chapter 4

Just How Benign Is the Natural History
of Low Back Pain?

The natural history of any disease or illness represents those manifestations and complications that occur in the absence of clinical intervention. What is the course of the disease or illness if simply left alone? Does it worsen or spread, or does it tend to be self-limiting and dissipate with time? An accurate understanding of natural history determines the gravity of the disease, predicts non-treatment results, and greatly assists in guiding both diagnostic and therapeutic decision-making. Understanding natural history is therefore imperative. Since the effectiveness of any treatment must be judged relative to the natural history with no intervention, "no treatment" becomes a useful alternative when designing randomized controlled trials (RCT).

Historically, with the absence of validated subgroups for most with low back pain (LBP), we are left with trying to characterize all of non-specific LBP as having a common natural history profile. By comparison, and not surprisingly, each different cause of chest pain has its own distinct natural history. Until we determine subgroups within the LBP spectrum, we are left with what will someday be viewed as rather bizarre discussions about the degree of seriousness of the symptom of LBP, again, as though all LBP was the same.

LBP's natural history is routinely stated to be highly favorable, with a 90% recovery rate reported within three months of onset. The European guidelines stated this 90% recovery occurred in as little as six weeks.[143] Acute LBP is therefore perceived as largely self-limiting; i.e., it resolves on its own, and is thus in questionable need of formal treatment. Such a benign natural history is a primary justification for current guideline recommendations for clinicians to simply reassure patients they will likely recover while encouraging them to remain active, based on some evidence that such care makes a difference.[143]

However, consider patients who have spent many weeks or months, perhaps even years, seeing clinician after clinician in an attempt to get relief from their persisting or recurring LBP and who would have been told at the outset, and perhaps repeatedly since (in compliance with guidelines) that the natural history of their LBP was good. No wonder they look elsewhere for care and patients are going in droves to alternative care methods in search of relief.

How often does recovery occur without treatment?

In a 1994 literature review of natural history data, in plenty of time to be considered in acute LBP guidelines produced over the past five years, Michael von Korff, ScD, senior investigator, health services researcher and epidemiologist at the Center for Health Studies in Seattle, Washington, and whose research concerns the natural history and management of chronic pain, pointed out that we had "great voids in our understanding of the natural history of low back pain," referring to our natural history knowledge as "incomplete and confusing."[145] He questioned the conventional "favorable" view, stressing the need for a better understanding of LBP's natural history to help evaluate whether alternative interventions are preferable to watchful waiting.

So just what is it that is so "incomplete and confusing" when clinical guidelines in no way equivocate that the natural history is benign? Let's visit the data.

One fundamental issue is that the evidence for the frequently quoted high rate of self-limiting back pain and recovery was derived from a 1966 study that never actually collected natural history data.[40] Instead, this study reported *care-seeking* data extracted from patient scheduling logs of general practices in the UK. When LBP patients did not return for follow-up, they were assumed to have recovered.

We can all relate to the response of Chavennes et al who, way back in 1986, cautioned that a non-returning acute LBP patient has not necessarily recovered.[24] There are obviously many other competing explanations for patients' non-return, including persistent pain that was not being helped by their GP. Care-seeking data is therefore a poor and unacceptable proxy for natural history. Guideline leaders are usually expert at recognizing such competing explanations.

von Korff based his skepticism of LBP's benign natural history on his report that 69% of recent and 82% of non-recent-onset patients were still experiencing back pain one year later.[146] He later published that 33% of those contacted one year after their LBP onset were still experiencing back pain of at least moderate intensity, 15% were still having severe back pain, and 20–25% continued to report substantial activity limitations.[147] These data would seem a more accurate reflection of these patients' natural history and also clearly portray a far less benign natural history than what guidelines continue to report.

In 1998, Croft et al reported the results of interviews with 490 LBP patients 3, 6, and 12 months after seeking care for their LBP.[35] His results were similar to von Korff's. Only 21% had completely recovered at 3 months. Interestingly however, just like the 1966 Dillane study, 90% had stopped consulting with their doctors by three months, further discrediting care-seeking as a surrogate for recovery. Even at 12 months, 75% of those surveyed indicated they were still not fully functional or without symptoms. A number of other studies also challenge the overly optimistic view of LBP's natural history.[26, 113, 142]

Meanwhile, the 2004 European Acute LBP Guidelines[143] perpetuate the assertions of previous guidelines by stating that "recovery occurs in 90% within 6 weeks with only 2%–7% developing chronic pain." How do these guidelines justify their portrayal of acute LBP as a benign health problem in the face of the von Korff and Croft data I have summarized?

More specifically, what evidence do guideline panels offer in support of their view? First, the European Guidelines offer no acknowledgement of the either the von Korff or Croft studies. They instead offer two references, neither of which is the 1966 Dillane study, but interestingly, neither of them are natural history studies either. The first is a 1988 article that presented no new natural history data[66] and only referenced a 1983 article that focused on some Swedish return-to-work rates after LBP.[8] While disability data are often viewed as a proxy for LBP natural history, von Korff correctly points out that we should "not confuse and make unwarranted assumptions about natural history based on administrative data on return to work or care seeking, neither of which are an accurate reflection of the natural history of back pain."[145]

The European Guidelines' only other reference is a textbook chapter entitled "The Epidemiology of Spinal Disorders" that presents a comprehensive report of data related to LBP prevalence, incidence, and risk factors.[6] I find no mention of the natural history of LBP in the chapter. The 1966 Dillane study happens to be referenced in the chapter but only for data on the frequency with which patients seek care from British general practitioners. Thus, not only do these guidelines provide no references that support their conclusion about the benign natural history of acute LBP, they continue to perpetuate the benign natural history theme that has historically been based on care-seeking data. Further, they ignore credible population-based natural history references whose data tell a very different natural history story.

So based on population-based LBP natural history data,[24, 35, 145-147] it would appear that acute LBP recovery is far less favorable than described in most LBP guidelines. Such an important revision in our understanding of this fundamental LBP characteristic has substantial repercussions in how we study and manage LBP. Doing little or nothing for acute LBP simply cannot be justified on the basis of such a favorable natural history, as claimed by most clinical guidelines.

Once again, as with the diagnostic triage, is this another case of expert consensus speaking its conventional views while ignoring relevant and conflicting data? Explanations for these discrepancies are unclear. The skeptic might refer to this as an example of Maier's Law: If the facts do not confirm the theory, they must be disposed of. Others might see this as the emperor wearing no clothes. Rigorous academics and research methodologists I have talked to have been far less kind in their assessment of this spotty and misinterpreted literature review.

But let's return to the second important natural history feature: recurrences.

Recoveries followed by recurrences

The second important characteristic of LBP, and where there is little controversy, is that it commonly recurs in the form of episodes. As many as 75% who experience their first episode of LBP have a recurrence.[77, 119, 142]

Although high recurrence rates are always acknowledged in LBP guidelines, they have oddly never recommended, to my knowledge, that clinicians impart this information to their patients. Is this tied to their optimistic view of the natural history of recovery, combined with an assumption that each episode is an isolated event uninfluenced by prior episodes, not unlike the common cold or a bout of the flu?[39]

Consequently, clinicians are encouraged to provide patients with the reassuring news of likely recovery but no mention of the high likelihood of their episode returning, often again and again. More complete disclosure to patients would seem the more appropriate, ethical, and accurate thing to do, and therefore something that clinical guidelines should be adding to their recommendations.

In contrast to the conventional view of a favorable natural history, true population data regarding this natural history prompted Croft to write: "The message from the figures is that, in any one year, recurrences, exacerbations, and persistence dominate the experience of low back pain in the community."[35] Full disclosure to patients should be the priority so they can make better health care decisions with their physicians.

Such disregard for the relevant LBP natural history data on the part of most guidelines is yet another factor in clinicians' lack of compliance with guidelines they view as consensus- rather than evidence-based.

We need to take this discussion several steps further

If recurrent LBP episodes were isolated events, uninfluenced by prior episodes, there would be justification in drawing parallels between back pain and bouts of the flu or the common cold.[39] However one recent workplace study reported that recurrent episodes led to more lost work time than first-time LBP episodes.[109] Likewise, both Croft and von Korff's data indicate that recurrent episodes often progressively worsen.[35, 147]

A 1973 study reported on patients whose pain had spread into their leg with a history of "acute stuck back" episodes.[41] It concluded that "these episodes are precursors to a disc protrusion since it is common in established disc prolapse to get a history of minor attacks of acute pain of this sort, with the symptom complex clinically reproducible."

Many studies have meanwhile concluded that a prior history of LBP is a strong predictor of longer or relapsing outcomes as well as the strongest predictor of a poor outcome with the current episode.[35, 110, 130]

Waxman et al conducted a three-year population-based survey concluding that recurrent LBP is "a mutable problem with acute episodes blending into longer periods resulting in more disability as time progresses."[153] "Most persistent disabling back pain is preceded by episodes that, although they may resolve completely, may also increase in severity and duration over time."

A recent analysis of 1,867 workers with new claims for lost-time from work due to LBP found that individuals with a history of recurrences had significantly higher total length of work disability and higher medical and indemnity costs than those without recurrences.[152] For those with recurrent work disability, 69% lost time from work, 71% had associated indemnity costs, and 84% of total medical costs occurred during the recurrent period. They concluded that secondary prevention efforts may be especially important. Doesn't all this sound very different than the common cold or flu?

Dixon also described way back in 1973 that many chronic LBP patients' prior recurrent episodes had become progressively longer in duration and more severe, until the latest one no longer recovers as in the past, and now has become chronic.[41]

In focused interviews of 349 LBP patients seeking care from physical therapists, chiropractors and spine surgeons, 64% reported previous episodes.[55] Of those, 55% described their current episode as the worst one they'd had so far, based on five parameters characterizing their current episode: 1) their pain was more intense than with prior episodes, 2) their LBP was interfering more with their work than ever before, 3) their pain was interfering more with their leisure than ever before, 4) prior episodes had never lasted this long, and 5) pain had never before radiated this far down their leg. Most reported that their episodes were worse by all five criteria. Despite the frequency with which these parameters for worsening episodes were reported, such questions have thus far never been asked in published population-based natural history studies. Having more data on the progression of severity over recurrent episodes would provide an important contribution to our understanding of the natural history of LBP.

If recurrences truly do often worsen over time, you would expect clinicians to notice this as well. And there's some data showing that they apparently do. In another survey, the entire group of family physicians attending a small general medical conference (N=33) participated in a paper/pencil survey that asked about their experience treating LBP, including their sense of the nature of recurrent LBP episodes. There was nearly universal agreement as to the high rate of recurrences. Further, more than half responded that, in their experience, recurrences commonly worsen over time.[54]

All these data beg the question that Dixon raised back in 1973:[40] does the underlying pain-generator responsible for recurrences deteriorate over the course of these recurrences to the point that it is finally unable to recover as in the past and finally becomes a non-recovering, chronic problem? If so, that would certainly be a credible, and perhaps even common, pathway by which acute LBP becomes chronic. Such a pathway might well be completely independent of any psychosocial factors to which the development of chronicity is often attributed.

One would then view the intermittent periods without pain (between recurrences) as a source of encouragement that the underlying problem is still capable of recovery. However, any worsening of recurrences would also indicate that the underlying pain generator is getting into progressively more trouble as it is repeatedly insulted. In how many chronic patients with a history of recurrent episodes has the underlying pain generator simply and progressively deteriorated to the point that it is no longer capable of recovery?

That worsening episodes are nowhere mentioned or considered in guidelines or in the thinking of most LBP experts could be explained on the basis of the existing lack of consistent data collection regarding characteristics of successive recurrent episodes in prospective population-based natural history studies. Most studies only inquire if patients have experienced prior episodes, with no further inquiries about whether they have worsened or not. These data will not be collected until there is sufficient appreciation that recurrences growing worse may move many patients progressively toward chronicity and non-recovery. But that first requires investigators to reconsider that recurrences could be relevant to both the natural history and management of LBP. The more fundamental question is: how long will it be before guideline panels will look at the ten-year-old population study data regarding the natural history of acute LBP to see that it is not nearly as favorable as currently portrayed?

Current data indicating that recurrences are not just benign acute episodes, but more commonly worsen over time, need to be examined as an important feature of the natural history of LBP. At the very least, there appears to be an important, even large, LBP subgroup in which recurrences may be an important pathway for acute pain to become chronic. Once again, not all LBP is the same.

Where does all this leave us?

To date, most LBP experts and nearly all LBP guidelines view acute LBP as a benign, self-limiting condition with equally benign, self-limiting recurrences being common. Chronic LBP, on the other hand, has been viewed as "the real problem," the expensive one, and one quite independent from acute LBP.

Many think that most physical causes of LBP would be expected to recover within 6–8 weeks, implying that most chronic LBP is therefore more likely due to some other mechanism, such as psychosocial factors.[151] Due to its high cost, chronic LBP therefore justifies intense study, with little perceived need to investigate such a benign, independent entity as acute or recurrent LBP.

What of the premise that most LBP commonly recedes or "runs its course" within six weeks? The natural history data I've just reviewed says otherwise. Further, if physical pain did persist, couldn't that be because the underlying pain source is not recovering for some reason? But what about chronic pain being mostly a psychosocial challenge? We'll return to that discussion later.

Contrary to the conventional view of LBP natural history, credible population study data indicate that the natural history of recovery from a current episode is not so favorable and that recurrences often worsen over time leading to more serious consequences than usually acknowledged. And this may provide a not so uncommon pathway to chronicity.

As we proceed, consider the following question: what if we could prevent a substantial amount of chronic LBP, including the need for some low back surgeries, by learning how to provide more rapid and higher rates of recovery from acute or subacute pain while also decreasing the high rates of recurrent episodes? The need for expensive treatments for chronic LBP would be greatly diminished and those out of work because of their LBP could return to the work force much sooner or, far better, they could avoid ever leaving work in the first place. Currently available scientific evidence that we will look at soon demonstrates that such improvement in LBP outcomes is not only realistic, it is already happening.

Chapter 5
Tackling Some Tough Questions

So are there any solutions?

Although there is no shortage of LBP clinical studies, including more than 1,000 RCTs, we still do not have satisfactory answers. But where do we go from here? What needs to be done? How do we avoid another 25 years of little or no progress in advancing our understanding and management of low back pain (LBP)? What can be changed on both the clinician and the research side of our Tension Cycle (Figure 3–3) so we can stop paying these extremely high and, in many cases, unnecessary costs?

First, we simply cannot make progress unless we are asking the right questions! Our main research question for the past twenty years has been: "What is the best treatment for LBP?" Addressing that question is the essence of the left side of our Tension Cycle where hundreds of RCTs have not produced any substantial improvement in the quality of our low back care or in reducing its cost. To the contrary, the management of LBP is still in turmoil, with the persistence of wide variation in care and increasing costs.

Current guideline recommendations leave payers few options in reducing their LBP costs. They either ration or completely deny some forms of care. But such tactics alienate both patients and clinicians while missing the mark as to how best to improve the quality of care and reduce costs.

So what are the right questions? All indications are that the right question that addresses both sides of our Tension Cycle, both the clinical and research components, must somehow get back to the fundamental issue: diagnosis. More specifically, especially with our limited knowledge of the anatomic source of pain in so many people, are there identifiable, distinct, and validated LBP subgroups based on patient characteristics and their clinical signs that respond best to specific and distinct treatments? Could there possibly be a new paradigm of low back care where treatment decisions are based on individual patient characteristics that reflect the nature of the pain source rather than treating 85% as though they all had the same benign problem?

The Tension Cycle also clarifies two other very pragmatic questions. On the right side, with all their extensive clinical experience, do LBP practitioners truly have little or nothing to offer 85% of acute LBP sufferers other than reassurance of recovery and encouragement to remain active, as most LBP guidelines would suggest? The left side of the Tension Cycle suggests an equally important question: Is there some fundamental defect or oversight with our past and current research strategies that has become an obstacle rather than a pathway to our understanding LBP and its management?

These are both critical questions that, not surprisingly, are closely linked. Let's consider this second question next.

PART 2
From Black Box to Classification-Based Randomized Clinical Trials: The Inevitable Transition

Chapter 6
Is There a Better Research Model?

The real purpose of the scientific method is to make sure Nature hasn't misled you into thinking you know something you actually don't.
—Robert Pirzig, *Zen and the Art of Motorcycle Maintenance*

The 1987 Quebec Task Force (QTF) proclamation that the initial step of making a diagnosis has been our "fundamental source of error"[132] didn't attract a lot of attention when first published, neither did it seem to affect clinical research activity. Perhaps clinicians looked to basic scientists and researchers for help while researchers similarly felt clinicians would and should be addressing this. But to this day, this "source of error" has remained the fundamental issue.

An international LBP consensus group published their list of the twenty highest priority LBP research questions in 1998,[14] identifying as their #1 research priority: "Can different varieties or subgroups of LBP (including chronic LBP) be identified and, if they can, what criteria can be used to differentiate among them?" Just like the QTF, this group also concluded that how we classify LBP patients is the most important question in LBP.

An article that same year from members of the Cochrane Back Review Group, another prestigious group of LBP research experts, stated that we should be performing RCTs of subgroups and emphasized the urgency of good ideas on how to identify homogenous LBP subgroups.[16]

Why is the identification of subgroups so important? Such an accomplishment would provide the basis for a windfall of productive research in at least six critical areas, in turn providing a much deeper understanding of the causes of LBP and its management.[14] Identifying and validating LBP subgroups would improve:

1. the objectivity of clinical decision-making (decreasing the high variation in patient selection)
2. the accuracy of outcome prediction
3. treatment outcomes
4. our understanding of disease process
5. the quality of our research design and interpretation of findings
6. the cost of low back care, dramatically

Clearly, the effect would be extremely positive, with valid subgroups providing access to a veritable goldmine of LBP knowledge. This goldmine will be the major focus of this chapter.

Another top ten research priority listed in that 1998 article was: "Is there a need for a new paradigm of LBP?" Do we need to, in some way, redesign our processes of low back care? We will address this question as well.

There were a number of other research questions on that top-twenty list that we will also be considering in some detail: "What are the best strategies for diagnosis?" "What are the predictors, determinates, and risk factors for chronic disability?" and "How can we improve self-care strategies and stimulate self-reliance among persons with chronic or recurrent LBP?"

Much like the QTF report ten years earlier, this 1998 article, although it listed so many important research frontiers, offered no answers or even any insights as to how to proceed in acquiring answers to these questions. It is my intent throughout the remainder of this book to directly address and answer these questions with published, peer-reviewed data; data that so many have overlooked or not appreciated. It is my sense that placing too much emphasis on randomized controlled trials (RCTs) has resulted in too many of us involved in education, research, and treatment missing the forest for the trees. It has likewise led to so many missing the elephant that is already in the room.

The Cochrane Back Review Group wrote in an overview article in

2003 repeating essentially the same message regarding the importance of subgroup identification.[15] In addition to describing their overall mission and work, they challenged clinical guideline convention by writing that "systematic reviews on the efficacy of preventive and therapeutic interventions can never provide an adequate basis for clinical guidelines." Ironically, most international guidelines seem to be just the antithesis of this statement. The recent European Acute LBP Guidelines actually state in their overall subtitle: "Based on systematic reviews and existing clinical guidelines."[143] How are we to reconcile those seemingly conflicting statements made by the world's most esteemed low back experts?

In this same article,[15] the Cochrane Back Review Group stated that, in addition to systematic reviews of *treatment efficacy*, "we clearly need additional systematic reviews of *etiological, diagnostic, and prognostic studies*." In other words, we cannot continue to limit ourselves to reviews of therapeutic RCTs, which have been and still are the mantra of most LBP researchers and clinical guideline panel members. This Cochrane article correctly pointed out the limitations of RCTs by stating that RCTs "can neither identify homogeneous subgroups of patients nor lead to promising new treatments." The authors further stated: "It may be deemed important to carry out a review of non-randomized studies in the absence of RCTs."

In my opinion, they have it exactly correct. This Cochrane Back Review Group has consequently initiated the development of protocols for the systematic review of both diagnostic and prognostic studies. Unfortunately, they acknowledge it will be 5–10 years before these protocols are completed and the first reviews are published. Meanwhile, it would be improper, if not unethical, for the rest of us, including clinical guideline panelists, to ignore existing non-RCT literature that focuses on these critical research areas.

Perhaps the most cogent statement was the Cochrane Group's acknowledgement of the importance of identifying LBP subgroups. They stated that determining "which interventions are most effective for which patients?" and "Which are the most important (preventable) predictors of chronicity?" represent the "Holy Grail"-type questions of low back pain. In modern-day culture of course, the "holy grail" is typically a metaphor for "the ultimate goal," while it also implies a distant and all-but-unobtainable goal. But does all this need to take 5, 10, even 20 years? Or could it be obtainable much sooner?

Have we been asking the wrong question?

We must acknowledge that the RCT is indeed the right design to answer the question "What is the best treatment?" But is this the best, or is this the only, question we should be asking? Is this where researchers, systematic reviews, and LBP clinical guidelines should be focusing? Not really. In truth, and based on what you've just been reading, most experts recognize that the most important question we should be asking is: "Are there identifiable LBP subgroups and how do we identify and validate them?"[14] It's just that so few researchers and clinicians are trying to answer that question.

Do LBP subgroups even exist?

There are some who even question the existence of LBP subgroups and feel that "non-specific LBP" may be as good as we'll ever get. Others, like the Cochrane Back Review Group, feel our ability to identify subgroups may perhaps still be far away, maybe even unobtainable; i.e., the holy grail.[15] Yet, as we discussed in Chapter 3 when describing the Tension Cycle, most LBP clinicians believe subgroups exist and at least try to make their clinical decisions based on their view of each patient's underlying problem.

There's yet one more irony: to my knowledge, no LBP clinical guideline has ever acknowledged the widely held belief that identifying LBP subgroups is a top research priority. Specifically, with only one exception which we will discuss in Chapter 7, no guideline group has reported on any non-RCT study designs in search of any evidence that LBP subgroups exist and how to identify them. Most seem to be content with, and even promote, the diagnostic triage, despite the lack of any evidence supporting its use.

How do we identify LBP subgroups?

How do we go about determining if subgroups exist and, if they do, how do we identify and validate them when we have such limited knowledge of the underlying anatomic causes of LBP?

A short review of reliability and validity

I have several times used the terms "reliability and validity" without explaining them. Many of you know more about these concepts than I, but, for others, it's worth a brief explanation.

Within the clinical domain, reliability comes in two varieties: intra- and inter-examiner reliability. Intra-examiner reliability means the ability of a single rater (typically the clinician) to be consistent in his or her decision-making. This is typically evaluated by asking the rater to evaluate an object, such as an x-ray, a slide under a microscope, or a patient's response to a physical examination maneuver, on at least two separate occasions. A number of methodologies attempt to keep these evaluations relatively independent in order to ensure that the object of the assessment itself hasn't changed between times of evaluation. When the rater is the patient and their response is to a self-report survey, this intra-examiner reliability is typically called test-retest reliability.

Inter-examiner reliability means the ability of multiple raters, again typically clinicians, to be consistent in their decision-making. Again, a number of methodologies and specialized test statistics, such as Kappa and intra-class correlation coefficients, have been developed to ensure that the way in which the information is gathered and analyzed provides appropriate estimates of agreement.

Consider Figure 6–1 showing Mr. Booth as he seeks another opinion about the cause of his LBP. After evaluating him, his new physician offers an alternative explanation for his pain—namely, that he doesn't have a slipped disc as he was apparently previously told, but his suspenders are just twisted. Such a diagnostic label would certainly qualify as one of those "inventive diagnoses" referred to by the QTF.[132]

Of course, this particular diagnosis requires the use of the "suspenders test" which, once one understands the difference between twisted and untwisted suspenders, is actually a test whose reliability is likely very high. In other words, with the proper understanding of the two possible test outcomes, if we all stepped behind Mr. Booth, we would likely agree on whether his suspenders were twisted or not. So the suspenders test would be quite a reliable test. If it were not, it would be a worthless test.

But while that simple "test" may have excellent reliability, it still may be worthless, for there is one more essential question that must be satisfactorily addressed: does the test have any validity or relevance to Mr. Booth's LBP complaint? After all, we might all be able to agree on his eye color or agree on his blood pressure with high inter-examiner reliability, but do those tests have any validity or relevance to his LBP?

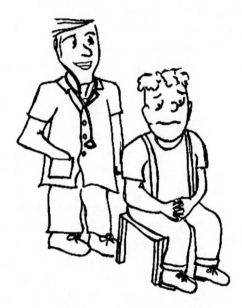

Figure 6–1: "You don't have a slipped disc,
Mr. Booth—your suspenders are just twisted."

Thus, although reliability is essential and necessary for establishing validity, it is not sufficient in and of itself. Validity testing is also necessary. One way to gain insight into the validity of the suspenders test would be to "correct" any suspenders deemed to be improperly crisscrossed to determine if the LBP resolves as a consequence. If it did in a simple cohort study, then an RCT of untwisting of suspenders vs. some other treatment(s) would be both indicated and justified. But, in reality, untwisting his and others' suspenders would likely have little effect on LBP. It is likely therefore that the suspenders test has little or no validity to his LBP and, on that basis alone, regardless of its high test reliability, would not a useful test for LBP.

The important message from this simple example is that both reliability and validity are essential before we can use and trust a test to help us establish the existence of a subgroup of patients or a diagnosis for which we might then begin to entertain some subgroup-specific treatment.

The A–D–T–O model: a classification-based research strategy

In one of the more provocative manuscripts written on the topic of LBP research, Kevin F. Spratt, Ph.D. not only evaluates and discusses the lack of progress in LBP research over the past 25 years, he then uniquely and constructively lays out a simple, logical strategy for addressing our need to identify LBP subgroups and determining more effective management over the next 25 years.[133] I've seen no other constructive contribution to the LBP literature that so clearly outlines the means by which we can identify and validate LBP subgroups. His coherent overview on this topic should be mandatory reading for all LBP researchers and for clinical guideline panelists as well.

As did the QTF fifteen years earlier, Spratt writes that the ideal medical model for patient care begins with the fundamental step of patient assessment which hopefully identifies a diagnosis for which a diagnosis-specific treatment exists that will resolve the problem. Clinical research, Spratt feels, should follow this same pathway in order to determine how to best treat individual patients rather than treating statistical means generated by RCTs targeting non-specific LBP.

He describes what he calls the "ADTO research model," with the letters A–D–T–O standing for "Assessment–Diagnosis–Treatment–Outcome." He emphasizes the necessity of scientifically and sequentially establishing each of the three research links between the four clinical components in this model (See Figure 6–2). These three links become the research building blocks that initially identify subgroups, which are later validated to have their own distinct subgroup-specific treatments. Following this A–D–T–O model requires the independent and sequential study of each of these three links:

1. The Assessment–Diagnosis link: performing an assessment and determining a diagnosis or descriptive subgroup.
2. The Diagnosis–Treatment link: for each diagnosis or subgroup identified, finding an effective treatment for it.
3. The Treatment–Outcome link: with the question of multiple diagnosis- or subgroup-specific treatments, which is the most efficacious? It is the RCT design that is used in establishing this third link, but only this third link.

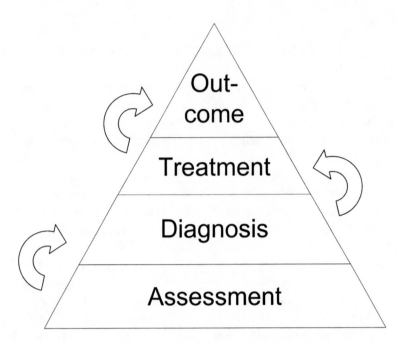

Figure 6–2: The Assessment–Diagnosis–Treatment–Outcome Research Model

"*The single most important thing,*" Spratt writes, "*is that establishing the validity of any one link requires that all previous links have already been established.*" In other words, it is inappropriate to jump ahead to the third, or Treatment–Outcome (T–O) link, that is, to conduct RCTs, without first establishing the Assessment–Diagnosis and Diagnosis–Treatment links.

Yet that's precisely what we've been doing for the past 25 years and our limited progress in identifying subgroups or efficacious treatments suggests Spratt is likely right.

Three essential research links

Let's look a bit closer at each of these important research links.

The Assessment–Diagnosis link

If each of the A–D–T–O links is a research building block, then the Assessment–Diagnosis link is the cornerstone in building our research project.

Let's be clear again that for most LBP, we are currently unable to identify an anatomic diagnosis. Consequently, the logical and best alternative is to identify LBP subgroups based on characteristic profiles derived from individuals' clinical presentations. Therefore, the "diagnosis" level of the A–D–T–O model is best addressed by subgroup rather than anatomic identification.

While discussing the Tension Cycle in Chapter 3, I pointed out that the high variability in classifying LBP patients was a direct result of the many forms of clinical assessments in use today, being taught across the wide spectrum of educational programs, most of which have no or little established reliability or validity.

Hence, the fundamental and first step, the cornerstone, in validating a diagnosis or subgroup is to establish intra- and inter-examiner reliability in determining if a subgroup exists and can be reliably identified. That is, can clinicians agree with themselves and one another on: 1) what circumstances dictate what tests or assessments should be conducted, 2) how to conduct these clinical tests, 3) the criteria by which a test is determined to be positive or negative, and then, based on those findings, 4) is there agreement on their resulting patient classification or diagnosis?

Most classification systems in use today have either never been subjected to well-designed reliability studies or have been studied and have already been found to have poor reliability. Perhaps the most prominent example of the latter is palpation; i.e., the use of the hands to feel and detect asymmetry, abnormal motion (often subtle) and/or soft tissue tension. Two systematic reviews have each concluded that there has been poor reliability with palpation across many published studies.[71, 123] Nevertheless, palpation continues to be prominently used by many manual therapists, chiropractors and osteopaths as a means of categorizing their patients. As we shall discuss further in Chapter 12, while it is often desirable and attractive to patients to experience "hands-on" care, the results from such assessments can be quite misleading and therefore even deleterious since incorrect conclusions about the underlying disorder are bound to send treatment down the wrong pathway.

Of course, establishing reliability in conducting clinical testing, interpreting imaging, classifying patients, etc., is a very challenging task. I predict that a number of subgroup classification systems in use today are unlikely to survive this initial Assessment–Diagnosis link in demonstrating reliability. When that is apparent, those systems need to either be revised in order to establish reliability, or discarded completely as unreliable.

Thus, the first and fundamental research step in moving us toward subgroup-specific care is establishing that a subgroup can be reliably identified.

The Diagnosis–Treatment link

Once a subgroup can be reliably identified, the second step begins the validation of that subgroup. A common way to establish preliminary validity is to first determine if members of the subgroup respond differently to a proposed treatment(s) compared with non-members of that subgroup. This can be done by comparing the outcomes of a cohort of this subgroup treated with what is hypothesized to be a beneficial intervention specific to that subgroup with the outcomes of those who are not part of that same subgroup but are similarly treated. A valid subgroup should demonstrate beneficial treatment results across multiple cohort studies. In this way, the case for investing valuable resources in an RCT focused on this subgroup is further strengthened.

Thus, such cohort studies of a valid classification system should not only lead to a distinct method of treatment for that subgroup but provide a reasonably precise estimation of the size of the treatment effect.[20]

The Treatment–Outcome link

Of course, the ultimate evaluation of the usefulness or validity of a subgroup test is to measure the utility of that test in improving clinical outcomes, that is, its efficacy. Since there may be more than one treatment that emerges from a variety of observational cohort studies as effective for a given subgroup, the best treatment can then be determined by moving to the final Treatment–Outcome link of the A–D–T–O research model.

It is only after the reliability of identifying members of a subgroup has been established (the A–D link), and only after outcome predictive studies show one or more forms of treatment to be potentially efficacious for that subgroup (the D–T link), that there is sufficient justification for investing the substantial time, money and effort to conduct an RCT to determine the most efficacious treatment for that subgroup (the T–O link). The A–D and D–T links are vital to informing the T–O link.

Some words of caution: just as in the past, it will continue to be the lack of focus on the A–D and T–O links when conducting future RCTs that will perpetuate the non-specific findings of the past 25 years of clinical LBP research. On that note, Spratt makes some provocative predictions: "Classic randomized clinical trials (RCTs), which generally focus on the treatment–outcome link without carefully and explicitly establishing the assessment–diagnosis and diagnosis–treatment links, are *doomed* [emphasis mine] because they leave too many alternative explanations or rival hypotheses for interpreting the results." He concludes that RCTs of the past have been "*meaningless, frustrating, and misleading* [emphasis mine]"[133] adding that "failing to move in these directions (toward the A–D–T–O research model) will result in articles written in another 25 years that suggest that Nachemson's (1976) lament,[106] that 85% of patients with low back pain have no specific diagnosis, remains as true then as it was 50 years before."

Consider this analogy

To illustrate Spratt's thesis, I have often used the following analogy to communicate both why our past LBP research has been so unproductive and why transitioning to this A–D–T–O research model is so important. Spratt used a similar analogy in his A–D–T–O chapter.[133]

You'll recall in my Introduction that I noted the absence of any "chest pain guidelines," for good reason. Let's return to the topic of chest pain and hypothetically suppose that we temporarily know little about the various causes of chest pain. Yet, in our efforts to treat those suffering with this common problem of non-specific chest pain, many treatments have been advocated and prescribed by various clinical interest groups. Not surprisingly, the wide variation in treatment and the resulting high cost have caused tension to resolve how to best treat chest pain.

In trying to address this tension, an RCT (hypothetical again) was funded that would randomize patients with non-specific chest pain to one of three commonly used treatments: nitroglycerin (NTG); an antacid (AA); and doing nothing, which serves as both a control and to provide insight into the natural history of chest pain (Figure 6–3).

When the data in our hypothetical black box RCT were analyzed, the chest pain of all three treatment groups had improved at followup, with a slightly better response using NTG or AA than from doing nothing, but no statistical significance.

With so little understanding of the pathology that produces all this chest pain, we must rely on statistical analyses to determine subtle differences in outcomes. So statistically, the difference between these treatment effects was so small that it begs the question whether the cost of NTG and AA justifies the little benefit they delivered compared with doing nothing.

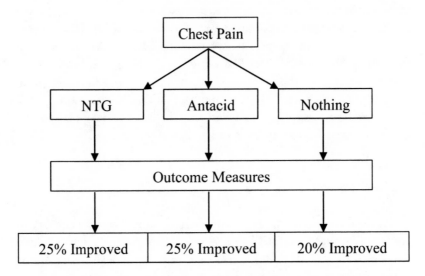

Figure 6–3: A hypothetical RCT of non-specific chest pain patients

Over time, this same black box RCT design is used to measure the effect of other chest pain treatments, with predictably similar and, again, rather non-specific results. The cumulative conclusion from all these studies is that "doing nothing" is as good, or nearly as good, as more costly interventions. Subsequent systematic reviews and chest pain guidelines would understandably conclude that there was insufficient evidence to recommend either NTG or AA in treating chest pain and that the evidence thus far supports that doing nothing is likely the most cost-effective treatment available.

So is this analogy any different than what has been going on with LBP for years that has essentially yielded similar "non-specific results"? It begins to be clear why so little, if any, progress has been made in improving our low back care, despite the incredible amount of invested time, effort, and multi-millions in research funding.

Fitting the analogy to the

Assessment–Diagnosis–Treatment–Outcome model

Let's shift our analogy to the point in time where research studies have identified a cardiac subgroup within the chest pain population along with some preliminary evidence that NTG may be helpful in this subgroup. That is, we have established reliability in identifying chest pain of cardiac origin with preliminary cohort evidence that NTG might be very useful in treating this subgroup. These studies now justify the performance of the identical RCT design with these very same three treatments (see Figure 6–4) but this time select only the reliably identified cardiac chest pain subgroup.

The results? NTG has now become highly efficacious in diminishing the chest pain of these well-selected patients. NTG would likely have been previously discarded for its lack of efficacy when investigated in the earlier black box chest pain RCT. Thanks to the A–D–T–O research process, the value of NTG now emerges as a valuable treatment for this large cardiac chest pain subgroup.

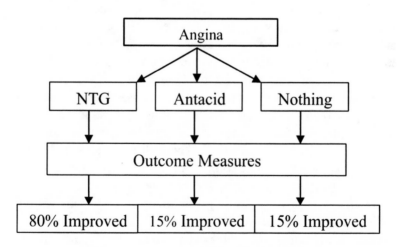

Figure 6–4: A hypothetical RCT of angina patients

As mentioned, such subgroup-specific studies add strong validation to this cardiac chest pain subgroup within the otherwise non-specific spectrum of chest pain. Of further importance is that the size of the non-specific chest pain group has just been substantially diminished by extracting the large cardiac subgroup from it.

Similarly, more A–D and D–T link studies would in time establish the reliability and validity of another chest pain subgroup: esophageal reflux. A repeat of the very same RCT study design and same interventions would then likely reveal that the antacid treatment would be quite efficacious for a sizable percentage of yet another chest pain subgroup. Again, a treatment previously discarded for its lack of efficacy for non-specific chest pain turns out to be of great value in treating a distinct and very common chest pain subgroup. And, once more, the size of that initial non-specific chest pain group decreases even further.

The dramatic difference when RCT subjects are selected on the basis of the A–D–T–O model clearly illustrates why so many research experts are calling for the identification of LBP subgroups. We return to explore the further benefits of identifying LBP subgroups in time.

But let's also look at subgroup identification in the context of patient selection for spine surgical procedures. Consider an operation performed on 100 patients with a success rate of 70%. No changes in the surgical technique and no new surgical technologies are required to substantially improve surgical outcomes if the patients with the 70 successful and 30 unsuccessful outcomes could somehow be accurately identified and predicted preoperatively. If so, we would only operate on the 70% subgroup, resulting in a hypothetical 100% success rate. Even a procedure with only a 30% success rate is still of great value to the 30% who did well. We just need to determine how to identify those 30% ahead of time. Much easier said than done.

Surgeons, of course, try diligently to avoid poor outcomes through better patient selection, yet there is an inordinate focus on trying to improve surgical results by developing new, and typically much more expensive, surgical technologies and procedures. There has been one new surgically implantable technology after another for the past 25 years and this process is even accelerating. Surgical specialists and spinal device companies so diligently focus on improving their procedures and very expensive technologies but continue to overlook the fundamentally important matter of patient selection, which is akin to researchers' excessive focus on improving the quality of RCTs while also ignoring the importance of patient selection in their continued efforts to study non-specific LBP, even to the point of ignoring existing evidence regarding how to identify and validate LBP subgroups.[78]

What about unnecessary surgery?

The risks and costs of low back surgery, such as surgical complications and re-operations, suggests that a high, and perhaps the highest, priority of all should be to avoid unnecessary surgery. Surgeons acknowledge this priority by routinely claiming that "non-operative care has been exhausted" before proceeding with any surgery. Typically, that "exhaustion" consists of some non-standardized progression of pharmacotherapy, generic physical therapy, and injections.

But does such a regimen truly exhaust conservative care? Are surgeons, and all other stakeholders for that matter, sufficiently knowledgeable about the full spectrum of available conservative care? The majority feel they are. After all, they operate on spines and know best how they work and what the pathologies are.

But are there non-surgical, non-invasive interventions that are specific to, and effective in, addressing the pain-generating pathology for which surgery is being contemplated? A fundamental question when evaluating LBP is: are there reliable indicators as to whether the underlying disorder will or will not recover without surgery? Can even those two LBP subgroups be distinctly identified? And can a patient, even though felt by one or more clinicians to be a surgical candidate, still *fully, even rapidly, recover* without surgery? If the patient can, it clearly suggests that some form of non-operative care has been overlooked by those who felt the patient was a surgical candidate in the first place.

My bet is that most of you are unfamiliar with three studies that focus on patients determined by their doctors to be disc surgical candidates and were on the verge of surgery that were then further evaluated and found to be members of a very important subgroup who could still recover, often quite quickly, when treated with appropriate conservative (non-operative) care. Now that's eleventh hour reversibility! But it also begs the question: why wait for the eleventh hour to provide that evaluation, unless it's very expensive (which it isn't)?

Patient selection: vital for both research and clinical management

Our chest pain RCT analogy illustrated that, despite using the excellent RCT design, a highly effective treatment like nitroglycerine can be completely overlooked as a direct consequence of poor patient selection for the study. Unless subgroups are reliably identified and preliminarily validated with prospective cohort outcome studies, continuing to perform RCTs, even with efforts to improve their methodological quality,[78] only wastes further valuable time and resources while perpetuating misleading conclusions as to what constitutes efficacious care.[133]

Besides writing that black box RCTs are "doomed" unless we first establish the assessment–diagnosis and diagnosis–treatment links, Spratt went on to say: "RCTs must begin with a very narrow focus, a single diagnostic group that can be reliably and validly determined, and for which a small number of standardized treatments can be justified."[133]

I mentioned earlier that the widespread use of black box RCTs has trained us to rely on subtle statistical differences in outcomes. For example, an area of great current interest and discussion in LBP research circles is: what constitutes "minimum clinically important differences" between group outcomes? Such a discussion becomes moot when studying validated subgroups rather than non-specific LBP. We can expect large differences in treatment outcomes when studying a subgroup, just as I illustrated in our hypothetical chest pain analogy.

Given the extensive call for the identification of LBP subgroups, a fundamental shift in our research strategy is needed. But when will this shift take place? Will it be slow and sporadic over the next 25 years, or can Spratt's message, and mine, help bring this to reality over the next five years?

Further thoughts regarding subgroup identification

Guideline panels' paradox

I alluded to this before but this point bears repeating. In determining their treatment recommendations, most guidelines have primarily focused on systematic reviews of RCTs which, of course, in turn evaluate the aggregate efficacy of LBP treatments for non-specific LBP, that is, black box RCTs. Routinely absent from guidelines is any review of reliability or observational cohort studies that would address the first two links of the A–D–T–O model. Again, this is truly a paradox. On one hand, many of these same experts are referring to the identification of subgroups as the #1 research priority in LBP, even LBP's "holy grail" according to the Cochrane Back Review Group.[13-15, 132] On the other hand, the very study designs that would address this high priority are essentially ignored by guideline panels in favor of their essentially exclusive focus on what Spratt calls "frustrating, meaningless, even misleading"[133] black box RCTs that emanate from the current consensus guideline classification, the diagnostic triage, which the European Acute LBP Guidelines acknowledge has no evidence to support it.[143]

Alternative research strategies for identifying LBP subgroups

An alternative research design envisioned by many researchers as the appropriate means of addressing our need to identify and validate LBP subgroups is to focus on diagnostic studies intended to identify the anatomical tissue responsible for the pain: intervertebral disc, facet joint, sacro-iliac joint, muscle or ligament, just to name a few. This is a real problem however, in fact currently an insurmountable one, since we have no "gold standard" test at this time. A gold standard test is one that is recognized as being able to identify with very high certainty what the true pain source is. The results of any other tests felt to have diagnostic value are then compared with the results of the gold standard test as a means for evaluating the diagnostic accuracy of the test of interest.

If we had such a test, we wouldn't have this huge non-specific-LBP subgroup with which we are unable to make a diagnosis. Consequently, with no means of identifying *anatomically based* LBP subgroups, this means of identifying subgroups is, for now, of little help. It is for this reason that we must look for subgroups by patient characteristics other than their anatomic diagnosis.

A competing explanation for our poor research progress

There is widespread recognition that our progress with LBP research is not what most would like it to be. Various views have been expressed regarding the basis for this poor progress. One view held by many research experts was expressed in a study of the methodological quality in design and execution of the nearly 1,000 RCTs investigating non-operative LBP treatments published since 1960.[78] With few exceptions, the quality of these studies was determined to be very poor across the board, with no evidence of any improvement in the quality of recent RCTs. No non-RCT study designs were included in the review.

The authors imply that it is this poor RCT quality that is the basis for our current uncertainty in efficacy of so many treatments. They call for much higher quality in future RCTs "to reverse four decades of inferior studies."

In yet another effort to improve the yield from LBP RCTs, these same authors, in another article, offered readers and study reviewers some insights into how to improve their ability to critique RCTs. They introduced a 40-item checklist for evaluating RCTs regarding their clinical relevance and applicability to the realities of patient care.[95]

Such measures intended to improve the quality of RCTs, while one cannot argue their value, fall far short of explaining the last forty years of inferior LBP research. The most perfectly conducted black box RCT will still produce non-specific results that are "frustrating, meaningless and misleading."[133] Gordon's First Law would seem to apply here: "If a research project is not worth doing at all, it is not worth doing well."

Evaluating current clinical approaches

Advocates and enthusiasts of most clinical LBP approaches usually claim their methods to be "evidence-based" when, in fact, there may be very little quality research to back up their claims. All clinical disciplines should be motivated to demonstrate or determine if their approach to LBP is valid. For them, the A–D–T–O model provides an ideally useful template for conducting new clinical research as well as evaluating the quality and value of existing research that might fulfill the requirements of the first two A–D–T–O links. We shall see, for example, that there are a considerable number of A–D and D–T studies already in place that have simply not been on the radar screens of systematic reviewers and guideline panels due primarily to their near total focus on black box RCTs.

A look to the future of research and guidelines

A crucial step in jump-starting our stagnant research is for researchers, funding agencies, systematic reviews and guideline panels to reconsider the currently elevated, but misplaced, role given to the RCT. The RCT needs to be removed from its place high atop its black box pedestal and relocated to its proper place at the top the A–D–T–O pyramid where it can perform far more productively as the culmination of a research building process.

Just as in our chest pain RCT analogy, we shall see later that by studying subgroup-specific treatments for validated subgroups, RCTs will begin to reveal more definitive, even dramatic, treatment efficacies.

Similarly, RCT funding should be withheld until these research priorities and strategies have been revised. Funding should instead be provided to support research efforts that focus on the A–D and D–T links, studies with far less overhead than an RCT.

Finally, as we have discussed and will revisit later on, in many cases, it is unnecessary to determine the anatomic sources of LBP in order to find valid LBP subgroups. To the contrary, as stated by Leboeuf-Yde et al, our search for anatomic causes of LBP will be accelerated by identifying LBP valid subgroups.[84]

The good news: an evidence-based pathway to recoveries and cost savings

Revamping our research strategy to extensively adopt the Assessment–Diagnosis–Treatment–Outcome research model might at first glance appear to take many years to sequentially study each of the three A–D–T–O links in order to establish the validity of any one LBP subgroup. That would still be such an important step in our progress over our next 25 years of research, rather than to continue our current research of non-specific LBP using black box RCTs.

The good news I wish to spread is that there is already published A–D–T–O evidence in strong support of how to greatly improve our treatment effectiveness while simultaneously and substantially reducing the high cost of low back care. This evidence and these methods are just waiting to be appreciated by a broader spectrum of LBP stakeholders.

In these next three chapters, we will look at what, for many, will be new insights into LBP and its management. I will be describing an exceptional and unique paradigm of low back care already supported by a substantial body of A–D–T–O literature established over the past 20 years. Failure by so many stakeholders to recognize its relevance to such a large percentage of LBP sufferers warrants both the writing of this book and you reading it. This is truly good news, both for those who suffer physically and those who suffer economically from LBP.

Let's get into the good news of the *rapid reversibility of LBP.*

PART 3
Good News! An Overlooked, Substantial Piece of the Low Back Pain Solution

Chapter 7
In Search of a Classification- or Subgroup-Based Paradigm

So far I have been attempting to create an important context for introducing a means of LBP management that is already re-shaping how we think about and care for LBP. This is a paradigm of care known and appreciated by only a relatively small percentage of LBP clinicians, yet they interestingly include members of an unusually broad range of health care disciplines who now value and utilize these methods of care. Over the past 25 years, many of these clinicians have said to me, "I finally found something I could offer my patients where I felt like I was actually having a positive effect on their back problem."

But it's only been in the past 15 years that these anecdotal stories have started to be validated by published research. We'll look at and consider that literature within the context of the A–D–T–O model in Chapter 8. To date, this paradigm has rarely been accurately portrayed in LBP clinical guidelines.

Some of you, hopefully many, currently unfamiliar with this paradigm will, after completing your reading of this book, recognize this as the breakthrough that it truly is. Many others already have some familiarity with this but are unaware of their significant misunderstandings that greatly jeopardize their appreciation for its value. There will actually only be a small minority of you who are already fully aware of the extent of the evidence in support of this form of low back care.

An evidence-based paradigm that starts with validated subgroups

Being absent from the forest when a tree falls
does not mean the tree never fell.

It's easy to ignore literature
never read or never understood.

"Mechanical Diagnosis and Therapy" (MDT) is the title increasingly used to describe a paradigm of care that has been best known for most of the past 25 years as "the McKenzie approach" to managing low back, thoracic, and cervical pain. These methods were first described by Robin McKenzie, a physiotherapist from New Zealand, in his 1981 textbook entitled *The Lumbar Spine: Mechanical Diagnosis and Therapy*.[101] It was expanded significantly in his 2003 second edition.[103]

Some may be interested, even surprised, to hear that there has been resistance amongst some leaders in the low back field to acknowledge this form of care because it carries the name of an individual. The most unfortunate outcome of that for so many is that the baby is then often thrown out with the bath water. If they don't like the name, the approach is ignored or denigrated. All this fuss despite the fact that so many diagnoses, surgical procedures, surgical instruments carry the names of the individuals who developed them.

But that baby is turning into the proverbial "elephant in the room" that many experts are finding increasingly difficult to ignore or pretend isn't there. We only see what we are prepared to see and learn from that which we are willing to read.

To begin with, let's be clear that these two titles for this paradigm are absolutely interchangeable: "McKenzie Care" and "Mechanical Diagnosis and Therapy."

Name aside, this approach has become one of the most popular means of low back care utilized by physical therapists around the world for addressing LBP.[9, 60] It is also one of the most common forms of care prescribed by physicians for their LBP patients. But despite being widely used by this clinical group, it nevertheless is significantly underutilized for the great majority of LBP patients seeking care from the full spectrum of LBP practitioners.

It also happens to be the most misunderstood, most misapplied, and therefore unappreciated forms of care, even by those who claim to utilize it. In research circles, it is very often construed as a one-size-fits-all treatment, specifically lumbar extension exercises. On one hand, this is easily explained by the long-standing research emphasis on LBP treatments and the T–O link addressed by black box RCTs. But such a focus completely misses the fundamental and essential element of this approach: patient assessment and classification.

Throughout the remainder of this book, I will be focusing on how this paradigm deals with LBP and the many important ramifications of how that contributes to our understanding of LBP. MDT is also very useful in addressing cervical and thoracic pain, but the scientific documentation for its validity in addressing pain arising from those two spinal regions lags far behind that published for the low back. However, based on both my own and many others' clinical experience and the research already published, it is strongly anticipated that a host of cervical and thoracic studies, similar to those LBP studies I'll present in the next chapter, will be forthcoming in these other spinal regions, with very similar results.

Given most LBP stakeholders' strong focus on LBP *treatment*, we should not be surprised that the most important and most often over-looked feature of the Mechanical Diagnosis and Therapy is its clinical assessment. The value of this assessment is that it routinely reveals valuable characteristics of each patient's underlying pain-generator. Read that again, for there is no need, fortunately, to identify the anatomic source of pain in most patients in order for them to recover. Yet being able to rapidly affect symptoms provides an excellent model to help both clinicians and scientists come to understand the physiological and psychological factors that actually cause, perpetuate, resolve, and prevent low back symptoms. As we shall see, it is the validity of this assessment in identifying relevant reflections of the underlying pain source that makes it so unique and so valuable in the field of non-operative care of LBP.

But before I get ahead of myself, clinicians and patients alike are often fascinated by a brief description of the origins of MDT and how it developed through Robin McKenzie's early years of ardent clinical observation and reasoning as he attempted to make sense out of observations with his own New Zealand spinal pain patients. Like most important discoveries, many years of observational science preceded the eventual published studies.

So let's briefly revisit this most fascinating story.

The origins of the McKenzie methods: a chance discovery with

Mr. Smith

The further backward you look,
the further forward you see.

— *W. Churchill*

Many great discoveries in medicine have been as a result of some accidental or serendipitous event. One of the best known was Alexander Fleming's discovery when he returned from vacation after leaving his culture plates unwashed. Something had "grown" on one of the culture plates that prevented the growth of bacteria around it. It was mold that was secreting a substance he later called penicillin which prevented these harmful bacteria from growing.

Many already believe that one of the most important observations in low back care occurred by accident with one of Robin McKenzie's patients, who he refers to as Mr. Smith. In 1956, Mr. Smith experienced an episode of acute low back and leg pain that then persisted over the next three weeks despite seeking Robin McKenzie's care. On arrival for one of his return visits for treatment, he was directed to an exam room and instructed to lie face down on the examination table to wait for Mr. McKenzie.

The room had just been vacated by a patient with a knee problem so the head of the table had been elevated for the reclining patient to receive her knee treatment. Mr. Smith complied with his instructions, entered the room, and lay face-down on the table to await his treatment (see Figure 7–1).

Five to ten minutes passed before McKenzie arrived to find Mr. Smith in this most unorthodox position. McKenzie was immediately concerned about his patient's well-being as this position was thought to be one to avoid for patients with LBP. Upon asking Mr. Smith how he was feeling, Mr. Smith reported that his leg pain was completely gone and he was only feeling some mild low back pain. "This is the best I've felt in three weeks!" he's reported to have said.

Perplexed but intrigued, McKenzie replied something to the effect: "Well, that seems to be working pretty well. I guess that will be all for today. Why don't you come back tomorrow and we'll try that again."

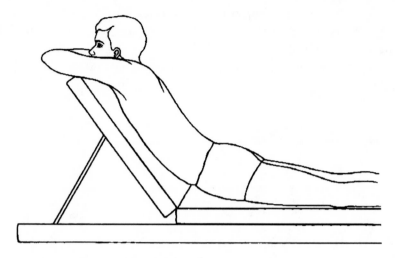

Figure 7–1: Mr. Smith lying in lumbar hyperextension for ten minutes

Upon arising from the table, Mr. Smith experienced no further leg pain. The next day, he reported he had only some back pain overnight, with no return of his leg pain. His LBP then completely abolished when McKenzie returned him to the same face-down, extreme back bending position (Figure 7–1).

Mr. Smith's unique experience both challenged and motivated McKenzie to explore the effect of this hyperextended position with other LBP patients. To his surprise, he found many who reported that, while they were lying in this position, their buttock or leg pain actually retreated back toward the midline of their lower back, a pattern of pain response that McKenzie soon labeled "centralization." The motivation to search for centralization became quite compelling since, whenever this response was elicited, patients usually experienced a rapid recovery, often accelerated by returning to this position at home if they noted any return of their symptoms.

With only one of these tables whose head could be raised, it soon became apparent that many patients could accomplish this same pain centralization effect by raising their chest up supported by their arms while letting their mid-section sag into this same hyperextended lumbar position (Figure 7–2). When their arms would fatigue before their pain had fully centralized, they rested by briefly lowering themselves, then pushing upward once again into the hyperextended position. For many, this repetitive means of extending their lumbar spine to its fullest extent, called "end-range" extension, proved easier, more convenient, and even more effective in some cases than trying to find a place or means of propping one's upper body as high as was needed to bring the same beneficial pain response.

This now familiar movement is used to both test and treat LBP with extension and is often referred to as a series of "press-ups."

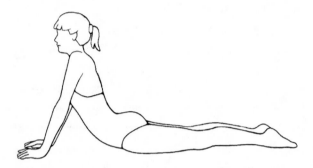

Figure 7–2: Prone end-range passive lumbar extension: the "press-up."
Performed repeatedly, this can be either a test or a pain-controlling exercise.

Of course, not everyone responded in such a favorable way. Such hyperextended lumbar positions promptly aggravated some patients' pain. McKenzie began to test other types of lumbar bending and found that centralization was experienced in other directions of bending; i.e., sideward lumbar bending or lumbar flexion. But interestingly, whenever centralization occurred, it was always the result of just one direction of testing.

Because of the substantial benefits of rapid recoveries by identifying a means of centralizing pain, a sequential examination evolved that has become the routine first step in evaluating and treating any new LBP patient. It made no difference whether patients' LBP was acute, subacute, or chronic, or whether it was only LBP or had radiated all the way to the foot. Centralization was found commonly in all of these types of patients. Patients with radiating pain would experience and report centralization and those with only midline pain could abolish that pain rapidly, once the proper direction of bending was identified.

This common finding, where a single direction of testing centralized or abolished the pain, later gained the name "directional preference."[52] Frequent repetitive exercising to the very end of patients' available lumbar range of movement in, and only in, that single "preferred" direction then became the patients' primary treatment intervention.

For most patients, their directional preference was lumbar extension. This was followed in frequency by lateral (left or right) testing, and was only found to be flexion in a small percentage of patients. It was this predominance of extension exercises, using press-ups and/or standing back bends, that unfortunately led many unfamiliar with this assessment to over-generalize and incorrectly conclude that McKenzie care meant treating everyone with extension exercises. To this day, despite the extensive writings and teaching about this paradigm since 1981, this misconception persists commonly worldwide.

I should add that a consistent finding of these patients was that their range of lumbar movement was decreased, sometimes substantially, when they presented in pain for their assessment. This limitation in movement persists in those whose pain cannot be centralized during the MDT assessment. But for those whose pain could be centralized and even abolished, the lumbar range of motion was simultaneously restored to normal. In other words, there was a consistent correlation between the range of the mechanical movements of the spine and the degree and even the distribution of patients' pain.

Part of any assessment is taking a relevant history from the patient. What became evident to McKenzie was how often a patient's directional preference could be ascertained from the patient's report of what positions and activities made their pain better or worse. The most common and clearest example was those patients whose pain centralized with extension testing. In their history, they invariably reported that their pain worsened with lumbar flexion: bending, forward leaning, mopping, vacuuming, working at a bench or sink, lifting and slouched sitting. They also reported their pain as better or even absent with walking or if they sat very erectly, both positions of relative extension.

Robin McKenzie has said: "Everything I know I learned from my patients. I did not set out to develop a McKenzie method. It evolved spontaneously over time as a result of clinical observation."[30]

McKenzie's most important contribution to our clinical examination

There's no doubt that McKenzie's most important contribution to the management of spinal pain has been the value of testing patients by having them bend their lumbar spines *repeatedly* to end-range, one direction at a time, in a sequence of mechanical testing, and to do so in both standing (loaded) and recumbent (unloaded) positions.

A common example of the importance of performing these test movements repeatedly is helpful here. Having a LBP patient perform a *single* standing lumbar extension test (see Figure 7-3) often results in a temporary increase in their pain. For many examiners, this alone suggests the likelihood of pain arising from one or more facet joints, the small paired joints located well behind the discs at each level of the spine. It is commonly understood that these joints are compressed or loaded with this direction of bending.

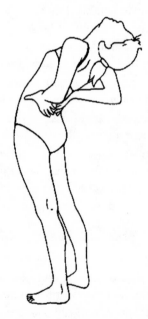

Figure 7-3: Repeated back bends extend the lumbar spine to end-range in the loaded standing position. This can be either a test or a pain-controlling exercise.

However, if these same patients perform this same standing extension test *repeatedly* to end-range, it is common for them to report the movement becoming progressively less painful while their ability to extend increases as they continue. It is also common that their referred or radiating pain centralizes to the low back until they only have midline pain and then that midline pain often disappears with additional repetitions. At that point, they have usually restored their full lumbar range-of motion (ROM) as well.

The results of only performing the single movement test would mislead many clinicians to conclude that extension should be avoided and the pain may be due to a facet joint problem, whereas it becomes clear with repetitions that just the opposite is true. It is quite unlikely to be a facet joint problem if repeated extension loading improves or eliminates the symptoms and restores full ROM. This improvement, which usually persists as long as the patient avoids repetitions in the opposite direction (in this case forward bending), strongly suggests there is something dynamic, changeable, improvable, *reversible* about the underlying pain-generator. Specifically, the pain source somehow benefits from a single direction of repeated end-range movements, most often extension!

A movement such as standing extension, that so often increases a patient's pain on the first attempt, if done repeatedly, will become easier and easier with the pain lessening, centralizing or even abolishing. This presents a very different picture to the examiner than if the movement had only been performed once. What is impressive is that the symptom location and ROM improves not only dramatically, but then subsequently remains improved after that direction of testing is concluded.

Obviously, the pain source is somehow compatible with the directional profile elicited. In a patient whose exam elicits centralization and directional preference, the underlying disorder has demonstrated its *rapid reversibility*, or its ability to recover quickly, as long as it is provided with the directional mechanical care it has demonstrated it needs.

Fortunately, the precise identification of the pain-generating tissue is unnecessary unless some invasive treatment is being contemplated. I say "fortunately" because, at present, the state of our clinical knowledge and technology provides no way to reliably identify and validate the pain source in the majority of patients. It is also reassuring that we can now characterize the mechanism of both the pain production and pain resolution in so many individuals without needing to make an anatomic diagnosis.

This examination is about mechanically challenging the pain source by loading the spinal joints and supporting structures while monitoring the patient's pain response for consistent patterns. These patterns provide a never-before-known window for gathering information about the dynamic behavior of each individual's underlying pain-generating disorder and what is needed to correct it. I've attempted to depict that window in Figure 7–4 by showing that this assessment process mechanically loads and stresses patients' anatomic pain source to reveal different patterns of pain response as well as prompt changes in patients' range of lumbar motion. This direct feedback from the underlying pain generator provides the examiner with insights into whether and how that pain source is affected by these standardized mechanical testing loads that comprise the MDT assessment protocol. We'll later discuss the breadth of this insight that enables the examiner to subgroup each patient, gain insight into their prognosis, and select their subgroup-specific treatment.

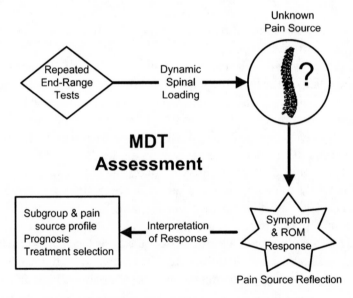

Figure 7–4: MDT assessment: the window through which
one can evaluate the pain source's response to mechanical loading.

So for most patients, the pain source and the symptoms themselves are quite dynamic, changing in intensity and location based on various loads applied to the spinal pain-generator, whether as part of the daily routine or a focused examination using repetitive end-range testing. But until McKenzie made and reported on his observations, we had no means of understanding or classifying the dynamic character of the underlying pain source.

For most patients, thorough directional testing also identifies directions that worsen their pain when performed repetitively. Those directions need to be temporarily avoided of course. But the good news is that in those same patients, there is usually a single direction of testing that creates lasting symptom improvement.

Of course there are some patients who report that these test movements have no effect on their pain, meaning their problem is not affected by mechanical actions. We will expand on this later but it is important to determine at the outset, using this assessment, which patients are and are not experiencing pain that can be successfully treated by using MDT methods. We will also see data that indicates that patients can be made worse if the wrong treatment is selected.

Treating patients with a directional preference

For this large subgroup with centralizing pain and a directional preference, treatment outcomes were so favorable and recovery so often rapid that a standardized examination emerged intended to exhaustively determine if some directional preference was present and, if so, what direction was it? These individuals' pain was clearly *rapidly reversible.*

The added benefit was that patients in whom a directional preference was elicited can then typically orchestrate their own rapid recoveries using directional exercises and postural strategies specific to the directional preference identified during their assessment. After the assessment, the clinician's role in securing the "cure" is largely educational, guiding the patient in their self-care. This obviously results in much less need for contact with the health care system and to much lower health care costs. At first, many clinicians have difficulty with the transition from providing the treatment themselves to merely helping and educating their patients to do so.

You can then see that this MDT paradigm of care is distinct from all other forms of care in that each patient's treatment is individualized, determined by the presentation and exam findings elicited by this unique assessment process. Treatment is not determined by a clinician's favorite treatment, and not by what school he or she attended or the discipline of which he or she is a member. Appropriately, the treatment is determined by the characteristics of the patient's underlying pain source. For treatment to be dictated by the nature of the pathology rather than the whims or biases of the clinician is obviously a preferred form of care.

As we proceed into this new century, given our continued inability to confidently identify the anatomic source of most LBP, it would seem that a new era in LBP management must be predicated on some means of identifying valid subgroups. MDT provides such an approach that empowers trained clinicians to characterize the nature and state of that problem or pain generator in such a way that in turn reveals effective patient-specific treatment. In most cases, it turns out, that is self-treatment that somehow directly affects that pain source in some beneficial, yet-to-be-delineated, way.

Indeed, this form of assessment enables the determination of whether or not the actual pain source is "reversible," an important attribute that no other clinical or high-tech imaging study has ever evaluated or even come close to delivering. Thus, although this assessment does not typically identify the pain source, it does determine whether that source is mechanically reversible or not, which in turn reveals all sorts of other valuable insights into the problem.

Three discreet syndromes

From the outset, McKenzie's experience using this form of assessment taught him that not everyone's pain centralized or exhibits a directional preference. Other pain patterns were observed however that reflected the presence of alternative types or subgroups of pain-generating pathologies. Again, it is quite logical that these distinctive patterns in which low back pain referred into the buttock and leg respond to what became a standardized form of pain response directly reflects the behavior and characteristics of the pain generator.

Three distinct patterns of symptom response emerged from his years of observations that led to three mechanical categories or syndromes. Members of each syndrome respond distinctively to these standardized directional end-range spinal loading tests that enables them to be classified into one of these three mechanical syndromes or else into a small "Other" grouping. Let's look at these syndromes.

The Derangement Syndrome, by far the most prevalent of McKenzie's mechanical subgroups, is what we have just been discussing in this chapter; i.e., centralizers with a directional preference. The term "derangement" is a common term in musculoskeletal medicine, meaning some disruption in joint articulation. A derangement's characteristic signs are that of rapid changes in both a joint's mechanical behavior and its symptoms, just as happens when a knee meniscus tears, often referred to as an internal derangement of the knee. In the case of a low back derangement, I refer to these changes as "rapidly reversible LBP."

McKenzie chose this syndrome's label for two reasons: 1) he had no way of knowing with any certainty what tissue was responsible for this syndrome so an anatomic label was inappropriate, and 2) the rapid changes in pain location, intensity, and range of motion these patients experience during their testing. Beneficial pain responses are very often elicited in the form of centralization and pain abolition while worsening patterns are also common in the very same patients when tested with spinal bending in the opposite direction. This means that the distal-most pain increases or moves even farther away from the back and down the leg; i.e., "peripheralizes." *The fact that one direction makes pain better and the opposite direction of testing aggravates the pain is the basis for concluding these individuals have rapidly reversible LBP.*

Like derangements in other joints, logic leads most to conclude that LBP commences and persists when something displaces or dislocates, and remains so until this displacement is reduced or corrected. As with a shoulder dislocation, patients first suddenly become painful and then remain worse after harmful mechanical stresses are applied to the shoulder and then just as suddenly improve and remain so after the joint has been reduced or returned to its relocated status.

So if lumbar flexion testing worsens lumbar symptoms, extension testing will usually centralize and abolish the same pain. Whether the patient then progresses toward recovery or not is determined by the amount of irritating flexion vs. beneficial extension forces that are applied each day to the pain generator.

Consistent with the disruption of any joint articulation, members of the lumbar derangement syndrome also typically report pain during their mid-range movements, more so than at end-range, so both the quality and comfort of their lumbar motion is typically disrupted.

Such a loss of lumbar ROM is often associated with an acute lumbar deformity, where the lumbar spine becomes painfully fixed in a bent position with considerable pain generated with most efforts to restore its normal lordotic curve. The most common deformities are usually in either a forward (kyphotic) or lateral (scoliotic) direction, the latter often called a "lateral shift." Even with these acute deformities, gentle end-range testing can still identify a means to rapidly improve the related symptoms, e.g. pain centralization, while simultaneously restoring the lumbar range-of-motion to normal as well. In fact, the loss of some lumber ROM is often the earliest sign of an impending recurrence of derangement, often even before any pain commences.

Patients with sciatica, including many with neurological loss attributed by most to nerve root compression from a herniated disc, typically meet the criteria for the derangement syndrome. It is here that the McKenzie assessment really shines, for no other form of assessment has the capability to determine (especially in such short order) whether or not the symptoms and signs created by a herniated disc are reversible or not. If reversible—that is, the pain can be centralized and even abolished with the proper direction of testing—logic would suggest that a means of improving or correcting that the internal nuclear displacement responsible for those symptoms and signs has been identified through loading the lumbar spine, and that disc in particular, in a specific direction of spinal bending; i.e., the patient's directional preference.

Again, McKenzie chose the label "derangement" for this group because these patients' pain was mid-range and acted like a joint articulation was somehow disrupted. When pain is centralized and abolished simultaneously with restoration of lumbar range-of-motion, it is as though something in that painful spinal joint has displaced and then remained so until this form of testing finds a direction of end-range loading capable of reducing or correcting that displacement. We'll get into this in more detail in Chapter 10. For those interested in treating LBP, it's a fascinating and provocative topic.

Let's briefly consider a patient who reports that her back and leg pain worsen with bending, lifting, and prolonged sitting. During her MDT assessment, her pain increases and even peripheralizes (worsens) as a result of performing repeated lumbar flexion tests but then centralizes and even abolishes her pain with prone repeated lumbar extension tests (Figure 7–2). She initially reports mid-range pain during her testing and limited extension range, but all these findings completely abate as her pain fully centralizes. At the end of her assessment, after performing repeated prone extension testing, she has full and pain-free lumbar extension as well as flexion.

By these criteria, her pathology would be classified as a derangement with a directional preference for extension. She would also be expected to recover rapidly, as long as her self-treatment consisted of frequent end-range extension exercises. Because both her history and exam indicated that flexion activities and positions worsened her, she must also temporarily avoid flexion, even though the ultimate goal of treatment is to return her to flexion activities with no symptoms.

In another scenario, some patients' pain is increased or peripheralizes with all directions of testing, includes mid-range pain, and would therefore also be classified as a derangement. But with no directional preference found, this would be an *irreducible or irreversible derangement.* This is a patient subgroup in need of further evaluation to better characterize patients' problems in hopes of determining appropriate treatment.

The Dysfunction Syndrome, far less common than the derangement syndrome, is characterized by intermittent LBP that is reproduced only when the patient moves to their lumbar end-range in one specific direction. They experience no pain when their spine is in its mid-range. Their pain is usually just midline LBP without radiation. These patients also demonstrate some restriction to their movement in that same painful direction.

The dysfunction syndrome is consistent with the presence of painful, adaptively shortened tissues that are the result of contracture or scarring from prior injury or surgery. These tissues are not painful until they are stretched by end-range bending positions and test movements. These painful shortened tissues also restrict bending movements in that painful direction. Unlike the derangement syndrome, producing this pain repeatedly by putting these structures on end-range stretch repeatedly does not make the pain change its location, worsen or improve as a result.

Effective treatment for these painful shortened structures consists of frequent stretching exercises several times per day over several weeks to repeatedly lengthen and remodel them so they no longer limit movement. In contrast to the needs of the derangement syndrome whose strategy is to centralize, abolish and avoid painful positions and movements, this group needs to do just the opposite: reproduce their end-range pain repeatedly to confirm that they are indeed stretching the painful shortened tissue. There's no rapid improvement with the dysfunction syndrome. Both symptoms and range of motion predictably are slow to improve. Recovery therefore takes several weeks of frequent focused stretching to enable the necessary remodeling.

Intentionally bringing on this pain during stretching is safe and non-irritating, as long as any pain from stretching subsides promptly (within five minutes) after stretching ceases. If the elicited pain persists longer, the stretching is too aggressive, tissue irritation is occurring, and one must back off the stretching frequency or intensity a bit.

The Posture Syndrome is an even smaller subgroup characterized by intermittent pain that is always limited to the center of the lower back and never refers or radiates elsewhere. It is produced only with prolonged positioning and loading of the spine at, or near, end-range, usually in flexion. Prolonged slouched sitting is by far the most common cause of this pain. The pain is typically abolished by the patient moving out of that end-range position.

Upon examination and repeated movement testing, patients with posture syndrome demonstrate no loss of lumbar motion, they have no deformity, and they feel no pain with any direction of testing. It is essentially a normal exam. It is only with prolonged time spent at end-range (i.e., in a slouched sitting posture) that the pain is reproduced.

Treatment is quite simple, consisting of education and posture correction that avoids prolonged time spent in the provocative end-range postures.

The "Other" subgroup includes those in whom one of these three mechanical syndromes cannot be identified after several sessions of mechanical evaluation. This subgroup comprises only a small percentage of the acute (of recent onset) LBP population and is more common in patients with chronic LBP. There are several small identifiable subgroups within "Other," including the red flag subgroup and those with dominant behavioral issues. Their distinguishing characteristics are described in McKenzie's text. For some, further medical review may be indicated.

These MDT methods of evaluation are conceptually simple but can in reality be quite complex to apply exhaustively, which is important to properly characterize each patient's condition. I describe the educational program and credentialing process in Chapter 13 as well as further information about this growing provider network.

MDT summary

Low back and radiating buttock and leg symptoms commonly respond in distinctly different patterns to both daily activities and the spinal testing of the MDT assessment. These patterns provide a window through which the mechanical characteristics and behavior of the pain source can be evaluated and characterized (Figure 7–4). It is obviously the pain generator that is being stressed as the patients' symptoms respond to these directional loading tests. If you can somehow improve the symptoms, you are likely providing benefit to the pain source. More specifically, if you find a way to consistently cause symptoms to move and change their location, you are very likely causing something related to the pain source to change its location as well.

Thus the MDT paradigm exhibits three important characteristics:

1. When low back and referred pain respond in any one of the three discreet mechanical patterns during this special form of assessment, it is reasonable to conclude that a mechanical and biological source exists, even if the patient's pain is chronic, and even in the presence of apparent psychosocial factors, a topic we will cover in some depth in Chapter 8.
2. Successful treatment and recovery from these forms of mechanical LBP does not require the identification of the anatomic source of pain. Yet even though we cannot identify the anatomic pain-generating lesion(s), since all the symptoms produced by that lesion or lesions can be centralized and even abolished, we can correctly say that the treatment determined by those pain response findings is therefore "pain source- or lesion-specific." This is difficult at first to grasp, yet it is a very attractive attribute of MDT: to provide pain source- or lesion-specific treatment without knowing the anatomic identity of the lesion itself.
3. Once assessed, the majority of patients, properly educated, are quite capable of treating themselves and eliminating their own symptoms and signs with patient-specific strategies. This is most often and most rapidly accomplished in derangements by empowering patients to first eliminate their own pain and then to either prevent or promptly and effectively respond to any recurrence of the symptoms.

"Half of what physicians learn
in medical school is untrue.
We just don't know which half."

Chapter 8

The Assessment–Diagnosis–Treatment–Outcome Model and Mechanical Diagnosis & Therapy Research

A scientific mind often begins simply with being skeptical of what it has been taught as "truth." Indeed, such skepticism is essential, otherwise a profession's traditions and dogma easily evolve into cultural idols without proper validation studies. Recall the idiom: "Half of what physicians learn in medical school is untrue. We just don't know which half." There's no reason to believe that doesn't apply to low back care as well.

The thinking of even the most experienced LBP scientists and researchers often evolves to where they become focused on only a very narrow view of back pain, producing minds that can become closed to considering any competing explanations or concepts. This process is no different than that which happens with clinicians who focus on one area of discipline in their training. While researchers continue their own diligent search for truth, they often do so only under that lamp post we spoke of earlier, whose placement is based on their own interests, biases, and dogma. They can see so much better under their lamp post, even though there may be considerable and valuable truths that, for them, seem to be off in the dark somewhere. The greatest truths may be underneath someone else's lamp post.

Robin McKenzie was originally trained as a manual therapist but was always skeptical of the reliability of palpation and the ability of most to develop the so-called "magical fingers" required for implementing that brand of spinal assessment. This skepticism was coincident with his experience with Mr. Smith which opened the door to what has turned out to be a whole new paradigm of low back care and an important contribution to our current understanding of LBP.

I have already mentioned the most common misunderstanding regarding McKenzie care: it is not just treatment, and it is certainly not just extension exercises. It is an assessment that classifies patients into distinct subgroups with distinct treatment needs. This misunderstanding is common in the literature and is even acknowledged in a 2006 systematic review pointing out that studies that do not include these assessment findings in determining treatment are really not evaluating McKenzie care, despite investigators claims to be evaluating it.[93b]

A brief review

1. Current LBP clinical guidelines recommend one-size-fits-all, non-specific treatment of acute non-specific LBP that consists of reassurance of likely recovery and encouragement to keep active while avoiding bed rest.
2. Guideline recommendations have not substantially changed either clinician behavior or the cost of low back care. Many clinicians view the findings of black box RCTs and subsequent guideline recommendations as irrelevant to their practice reality of treating individual patients.
3. To deal with the incongruence between guideline recommendations and clinicians' practice patterns, the A–D–T–O clinical research strategy model has been proposed that first seeks to reliably identify LBP subgroups that can then be validated using outcome predictive cohorts and finally subgroup-focused RCTs. Discontinuing "black box" RCTs all together is an important consideration.

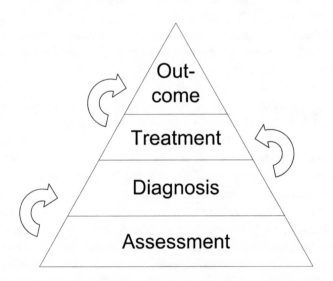

Figure 8–1: The Assessment–Diagnosis–Treatment–Outcome Research Model

4. The McKenzie/Mechanical Diagnosis and Therapy (MDT) methods of low back care are unique because they commence with a standardized clinical assessment enabling the identification of distinct mechanical pain responses that must in some way directly reflect the presence or absence of one or more distinct types of mechanical pain generator, each of which has its own subgroup-specific treatment protocol. In other words, the most appropriate treatment for each individual patient is guided by each patient's pattern of pain response that emerges during his or her assessment.

5. The elimination of the pain is typically best carried out by patients themselves, and, once patients are educated and empowered to do so, can very often be done quickly. This characteristic of *rapidly reversible* symptoms is not widely appreciated.

"So what!"

"So is MDT any different, or any better, than any other treatment?" you ask. "I've known about McKenzie care for a long time. Where's the evidence that validates it and, if it's so good, why are we not reading more about it in the systematic reviews and clinical guidelines?"

It has in fact been acknowledged in some guidelines as a useful treatment.[97, 112] But as you realize by now, one of the biggest reasons is that most every RCT has defined it as extension exercises, as has every international clinical guideline thus far, but one.[97] They have all focused only on black box RCTs, ignoring the growing body of evidence regarding the ability of the MDT assessment to identify valid LBP subgroups.

The single exception is the Danish acute LBP guidelines published in 1999.[97] It is the only guideline to review studies pertaining to the MDT assessment process. With only the limited evidence available prior to 1999, these guidelines uniquely concluded: "the (McKenzie) method has value as both a diagnostic tool and a prognostic indicator." "This technique can be recommended as a diagnostic method for both acute and chronic pain syndromes." In fact, they assigned their second highest grade for scientific evidence in support of the diagnostic value of the McKenzie assessment procedures.

So where is that evidence and why aren't other guidelines recognizing it?

The Danes were subsequently criticized by members of other guideline panels over their McKenzie recommendations based on those panels' views that insufficient treatment effect exists while completely ignoring all the literature that evaluates the assessment process. Is this a case of: *"I don't understand how this works, therefore it doesn't exist"*?

Please note that the Danish Guidelines also addressed the McKenzie *treatment* methods, stating that "McKenzie exercises can be considered as a treatment method for both acute and chronic low-back pain." They however correctly did not give McKenzie *treatment* as high a grade as they did for McKenzie *assessment* based on the insufficiency of the treatment evidence at that time. Thus, most guideline panels continue to focus on evaluating outcomes and ignore evaluating the quality of the process of assessing patients for the purposes of classifying or diagnosing them and, in so doing, they have solidly placed the cart before the horse. It is unclear why they would do this, given that the identification of subgroups is so widely advocated.

As we shall now see, there are many non-RCT studies that evaluate this classification process and how to identify and validate LBP subgroups. They are simply being ignored by LBP experts who justify their view by persisting in asking what they feel is the ultimate question: "What is the best treatment for LBP?"

How does the Assessment–Diagnosis–Treatment–Outcome model help us here?

Within the A–D–T–O model, the required studies for the first two links are not RCTs, which is why these studies have remained under the radar for nearly all LBP guidelines, which historically have limited their literature reviews to RCTs. So let's now return to the A–D–T–O model as our template in reviewing and evaluating the existing literature pertaining to these MDT methods of care.

The studies referenced in the remainder of this chapter are summarized in the Appendix.

The Assessment–Diagnosis link

This 1987 Quebec Task Force statement is worth re-reading: "There is so much variability in making a diagnosis that this initial step routinely introduces inaccuracies which are then further confounded with each succeeding step in care."[132] Spratt then, in 2002, took this same theme one step further by stating: "Variability in diagnosis falls at the feet of invalid assessment."[133]

In Chapter 6, we discussed that the first step in classifying patients into subgroups, and reducing variability when conducting a clinical exam, is establishing intra- and inter-examiner reliability; i.e., the Assessment–Diagnosis, or the A–D link of the A–D–T–O research model.

Although insufficient attention has been given to reliability studies overall, they are fundamental to the whole clinical research process. Validity cannot exist without first establishing adequate reliability.

Nikolai Bogduk, MD, Ph.D., DSci., is a well published researcher and Professor of Pain Medicine at the University of Newcastle in Newcastle, Australia. He is known for being brutally honest in his critique of the quality of evidence pertaining to any diagnostic or treatment intervention. He accepted the invitation to write the Foreword for the 2003 edition of McKenzie's lumbar textbook[103] in which he stated that MDT's "reliability is now beyond doubt" but noted it "is contingent upon training. Although anyone can assess according to the system, it cannot be mastered by hearsay or assumption." On what is he basing these statements?

No form of LBP clinical assessment has been investigated for its reliability as extensively as the MDT assessment protocols and classification. To date, at least nine such studies have been published that were unanimous in reporting good-to-excellent reliability (Kappa values ranging from .79 to 1.0) when using examiners who are "credentialed" by the McKenzie Institute.[30, 31, 64, 75, 76, 116, 134, 158, 161] Again, we'll discuss what "credentialing" means in Chapter 13. Some of these studies targeted the reliability of the specific findings of the repeated end-range movement tests while others showed strong reliability in classifying patients into diagnostic subgroups based on theses exam findings.

Two other studies are noteworthy for their report of only fair or poor reliability for centralization and/or MDT subgroups, but both studies used examiners who had little, if any, formal training in MDT, as taught by the McKenzie Institute.[62, 117]

One of these is part of a series of studies that address a very interesting system of LBP management best known as "the Delitto treatment-based classification system." It also recognizes centralization as the basis for one of the three main categories of LBP and so eliciting centralization is an important objective of its initial assessment.[65] This paradigm of care then appropriately prescribes directional exercises as treatment for this centralization subgroup. To date, only testing in the sagittal plane, that is flexion and extension, is included in their assessment, with no indication in the literature that directional education such as posture modifications are included in the treatment of this subgroup. The assessment and treatment of this subgroup in this Delitto system continues to evolve however.

These researchers have also appropriately conducted reliability studies targeting the ability of practitioners to classify patients into their three subgroups. Their reliability in identifying their various subgroups varies depending upon the subgroup. Their reliability in identifying centralization has so far not been strong (Kappa = .15 to .55).[62, 65] Thus, to date, the reliability studies that report high Kappa values are those using the MDT assessment conducted by clinicians who have been trained and credentialed through the McKenzie Institute.[30, 31, 76, 116, 158] MDT training is readily available to members of all clinical disciplines through the McKenzie Institute (see Chapter 13).

One study merits further comment because of the high reliability it reported in identifying centralization, yet it also concludes that such high reliability occurs even with non-McKenzie trained P.T. students.[64] This suggests of course that expertise is not a requirement for reliably identifying centralization. However, the study did not evaluate examiners' ability to *elicit* centralization, only to identify it on video when a patient said his or her pain moved proximally. I would contend that little if any training is required to recognize when a patient states their pain has changed location. But the issue of expertise lies in the ability to elicit the centralization response and classify patients accordingly. Another study meanwhile demonstrated that poorly trained clinicians were unreliable in eliciting pain responses and classifying patients[117] and at least five other studies have uniformly shown reliability with clinicians who have attained the Credentialed level of proficiency or higher.[30, 31, 76, 116, 158]

One further note: one would also naturally expect that variations in training would lead to differences in the reported prevalence of centralization and directional preference. In studies reporting low prevalence, one would then need to question whether any centralizers are being missed as opposed to being overcalled in high prevalence studies. It is in fact the high reliability studies that report high centralization prevalence while the low reliability studies report lower rates of centralization. It is also the high prevalence studies that all strongly report both good outcomes for the centralization subgroup and poor outcomes for non-centralizers. It seems unlikely therefore that the high prevalence rates are over-identifying centralization.

What remains to be seen is what adjustments will be made by practitioners of this treatment-based system in lieu of their low reliability in eliciting and identifying centralization. Many feel that their reliability testing should be repeated using clinicians who are credentialed in MDT. This should not be difficult. Collaborative research between the two clinical systems of MDT and Delitto would be extremely enlightening.

Good reliability has of course also been shown for some non-MDT testing, including manual tests that rely on patients' report of pain provocation.[83, 98, 114, 139] But without the pain provocation element of testing, palpation has otherwise been shown to be unreliable, as reported in two separate systematic reviews.[71, 123] For those unfamiliar with palpation, it is the use of the examiner's hands to feel and detect asymmetries or abnormalities in anatomic landmarks and spinal and pelvic movements.

Reliability is an important issue because manual palpation without pain provocation remains a staple in the evaluation methods of large LBP clinician groups. Many chiropractors, manual therapists, osteopathic physicians and massage therapists continue to rely heavily on palpation for their clinical evaluation, but the lack of reliability greatly undermines the objectivity of their decision-making efforts to draw valid conclusions from their assessment.

Fortunately, a small but growing number of leaders in these manual disciplines are acknowledging this unreliability. Some are striving to find ways to show the reliability of certain forms of palpation while others are finding MDT assessment methods to be very satisfying and an informative part of their initial patient evaluation. Thus pain provocation, in many forms, has proven to be very reliable and an important part of clinical testing, whether part of manual testing or patient self-testing with repeated end-range movements as in the MDT assessment methods. It is also worthwhile noting that most of the traditional and widely used clinical tests for LBP are also pain-provocation tests. Two such tests involve pain increase as the endpoint of the test: the straight-leg-raising test and measuring lumbar range-of-motion. Even Waddell tests for signs of non-organic features use non-organic symptom reporting to determine the outcome of the tests.[150]

With such strong reliability evidence for identifying centralization, directional preference, and derangements, the Assessment–Diagnosis link for this large clinical subgroup, despite our inability to make an anatomical or tissue diagnosis, is already well-established for the MDT methods.

The Diagnosis–Treatment link

Once the A–D link is established, one is then able to focus on the Diagnosis–Treatment (D–T) link. Just like with the twisted suspenders test, the D–T research question becomes: Is there evidence that this centralization/directional preference subgroup has any relevance or validity to the patient's LBP complaint? And, is there a treatment for centralizing/directional preference patients that will alleviate their low back complaint?

At the most fundamental level, the relevance or validity of centralization to low back and referred pain is unquestionable. How could it be otherwise? How could it be invalid or irrelevant when it defines the behavior of the very symptom we are investigating and for which the patients are seeking care? Thus, the "face" validity of MDT between diagnosis and treatment is obvious. But this form of validity in the measurement world is felt to be the weakest form of validity evidence. In the clinical world however, without strong face validity, few are willing to look any deeper.

A more substantial form of validity is *construct validity*[24], which, within the D–T link, establishes that those treated in a proposed subgroup-specific way do better than those in different subgroups given the same treatment and better than those in the same subgroup given a different treatment.

But we must be careful at this point not to jump the gun by focusing too early on finding *the best* treatment. That is left for the Treatment–Outcome link, where RCTs provide the best means for evaluating treatment efficacy. In the D–T link, we are merely looking to identify best treatment candidates for a reliably identified subgroup. Longitudinal cohort and observational studies are quite adequate in establishing the D–T link.

Prevalence of directional preference and centralization

An important feature of such cohort series is the opportunity to determine the prevalence of a subgroup within the whole non-specific-LBP population. Of course, the higher the prevalence, the more prominent and important the subgroup, pending the outcomes of D–T and T–O links. Obviously, the size of the non-specific-LBP population diminishes proportionally with the identification and validation of each subgroup.

The initial centralization study published in 1990[56] reported that the radiating pain of acute LBP centralized during an MDT assessment 87% of the time. The prevalence was nearly as high in those in pain for over three months. These were consecutive LBP adults with pain radiating into their thigh or lower, who presented to my orthopedic practice for care.

Since 1990, at least ten other studies have reported on the high prevalence of centralization and directional preference in their study populations.[37, 50-52, 56, 72, 82, 88, 90, 129, 136, 158] Overall, reported prevalence has been 70–87% across acute LBP studies and in 32–52% of patients with chronic LBP.

A very important point arises here. With such a high prevalence reported in so many studies, if the centralization/directional preference subgroup proves its validity in subsequent D–T and T–O studies, then this large subgroup should become a prime target of all sorts of investigations, which we will discuss later.

Predicting treatment outcomes for those who exhibit centralization and directional preference

In the MDT paradigm of care, once a single beneficial direction of movement (i.e., the patient's directional preference) is reliably identified, patients are instructed in self-treatment, specifically regarding when and how to correctly perform simple yet precise end-range directional exercises several times a day, while temporarily avoiding movements or positions that take the lumbar spine in the opposite direction, that is postural strategies, thereby temporarily avoiding that direction of lumbar bending that re-produced or aggravated their pain in their history and during testing.

The centralizers in that 1990 cohort study of acute LBP reported good or excellent recoveries at a very high rate (98%) at the time of discharge from care. Although not reporting any long term follow-up, these recoveries were obviously both far more numerous and far quicker than any other competing explanation might predict (such as recovery by natural history or regression to the mean).

Since that first centralization study, at least seven other cohort studies have unanimously reported that basing treatment strategies on individual patients' MDT exam findings produced good or excellent outcomes for both acute and chronic patients.[56, 65, 72, 88, 90, 129, 136, 157, 158] Several of these studies also reported on patients in whom a directional preference could not be elicited and who consistently had very slow recoveries, or even non-recovery. Werneke, for example, reported that acute patients found at baseline to be centralizers had good and excellent outcomes at one year but that non-centralizers had a stronger chance of experiencing prolonged or non-recoveries.[157, 158]

Please be clear that the directional preference/centralizing patients in every one of these studies were treated by well-trained MDT clinicians. As such, each patient's treatment was individualized, determined by his or her specific assessment findings. It is also important to realize that, by not being RCTs, none of these studies determined if the consistently good outcomes for this subgroup require this specific treatment or whether this subgroup would experience good outcomes regardless of treatment.

Consequently, despite such a very high success rate with this form of care, we need to address whether this MDT assessment is merely identifying those with an excellent prognosis independent of how they are treated, or if the treatment that matches their assessment findings is an essential piece to their successful outcomes?

Only an RCT design can answer these questions, which is the next and final step in the A–D–T–O research protocol. But we should acknowledge that there is already ample evidence to establish at least preliminary validation of centralization and directional preference, so at least the D–T link for the centralization/directional preference subgroup is firmly established.

We now have sufficient evidence to establish both the A–D and D–T links for MDT

Dr. Alf Nachemson, a highly respected authority on LBP for many decades, in his somewhat bombastic style so familiar to those who have heard him speak, loudly and emphatically announced during one of his podium presentations at an international spine conference a few years ago: "We don't need any more studies to prove that too much bed rest is not good."

It would not be inappropriate to respond similarly today regarding the prevalence, reliability and prognostic studies for centralization and directional preference. We don't need any more of these studies. Multiple studies and systematic reviews document that centralization and directional preference are highly prevalent.[37, 50-52, 56, 72, 82, 88, 90, 129, 136, 158] Multiple studies also document that centralization and directional preference are reliably identified when clinicians are adequately trained.[30, 31, 64, 75, 76, 116, 134, 158, 161] Finally, these same clinical findings have been shown in multiple studies to predict highly successful outcomes if patients are treated accordingly.[56, 65, 72, 88, 90, 129, 136, 157, 158]

The Treatment—Outcome link

With the first two A–D–T–O links well-established, we are now justified in investing time, effort, and great expense of conducting an RCT targeting this centralization/directional preference subgroup. As we illustrated in our hypothetical chest pain RCT in Chapter 6, by focusing an RCT on a preliminarily validated subgroup, one can have high expectations that the RCT will produce some important positive findings, even dramatic ones, of far greater significance and value than what have so routinely emerged from the hundreds of past "black box" RCTs.

Subgroup-specific RCTs

The research question: Would centralizing/directional preference patients have the same excellent recoveries if treated some non-MDT way? Does it really matter how this subgroup is treated or would they do just as well if treated with the one-size-fits-all care recommended by current guidelines? What is the best treatment for this subgroup? Showing that outcomes for this subgroup are improved as a result of identifying this subgroup is the ultimate test of validity.

There are now four RCTs targeting centralization/directional preference that directly address these questions. The first was a small study in 25 patients with LBP and radiculopathy who were found at baseline to be members of "the derangement subgroup."[121] You'll remember that's the McKenzie syndrome that is characterized by patients found to have a directional preference and be centralizers. These patients were then randomized to either directional exercises selected on the basis of their directional preference findings (N=15) or to manual techniques selected on the basis of findings from an assessment that uses active and passive intervertebral motion testing (N=10). Subjects were only followed over their course of three physical therapy visits. In that short time, those treated with McKenzie exercises reported a significantly greater decrease in pain level (p<.01) and improvement in function (p<.03) compared to the manual mobilization group. But such a small sample has little generalizability to the non-specific-LBP population.

The second RCT by Long, et al is a different story.[90] One of this study's many strengths is its great generalizability since amongst its 230 subjects were not only patients with acute, subacute, and chronic conditions but those whose pain location and neurological status were also quite diverse. About one-half had LBP-only, while 34% had full leg pain (sciatica) and half of those had a mild neurological loss.

Like the first study, only those found to have directional preference during an initial MDT assessment were included in the study. These directional preference patients were then randomly assigned to treatment with either directional exercises that "matched" their directional preference (MDT) or to one of two "unmatched" exercise programs. One of these two latter programs prescribed exercises in the direction opposite to their directional preference while the other provided evidence-based care resembling recent guideline recommendations of assurance, advice, and education to keep active, as well as a general non-directional exercise program.

As in prior cohort studies, the prevalence of directional preference was high, found in 74% of the 312 consecutive patients that presented in the eleven low back clinics who participated in this study. After just two weeks of treatment, while the statistical means of all three treatment groups showed improvement, patients treated with directional preference-specific or matching-directional exercises reported dramatically greater improvement in all seven of the study's outcome measures (back and leg pain, physical function, medication use, self-report of degree of recovery, activity interference, and depression). These improvements were hardly subtle, ranging from two to five-fold gains for the matched exercise group compared with the outcomes of subjects treated with either of the two unmatched exercise programs.

Of those in the matching exercise/MDT treatment group, 95% reported being either better or fully recovered at two weeks. This was more than twice the 42% with similar results in the Evidence-Based Care group and more than four times the 23% in the Opposite direction exercise group. In fact, one-third of patients treated in either of the unmatched exercise groups withdrew from the study before two weeks due to being either worse or no better. Of particular importance, 15% of both the non-matching treatment groups actually reported being worse compared with no subject in the matched exercise group reporting worsening.

Interestingly, this 95% improvement in the matching exercise treatment group agreed with the 95% recovery rate in the very first centralization cohort study published in 1990.[56]

This study addressed the very important question we asked earlier: since centralizing/directional preference patients have reported such good outcomes in so many prior cohort studies, does it matter how directional preference patients are treated? These data indicate that it definitely does matter. Those receiving directional preference-specific treatment (matching directional exercises) did dramatically better. In fact, despite the excellent prognosis expected from so many cohort studies for patients exhibiting a baseline directional preference, 15% of both of the unmatched treatment groups were actually made worse.

Special attention should be focused on the report that evidence-based treatment (advice to stay active, reassurance, gentle mid-range activity and exercise), the very care recommended by every LBP clinical guideline, actually worsened 15% of the patients who were strongly predicted and expected to do well.

These results are not subtle, which has become the widespread expectation from black box RCTs to date. But these dramatic results should also not be a total surprise, if we recall our hypothetical chest pain RCT analogy (Chapter 6) that compared the non-specific results of a black box RCT with the much more impressive outcomes in the cardiac subgroup RCT.

It is important to understand that this study, in and of itself, is not about a cure for LBP. Two weeks of follow-up is insufficient to evaluate the long-term benefits. But there are other studies that document the long-term benefits of treating centralizers and directional preference patients with matching exercises and posture strategies.[111, 158] This study is about the rapid and significant effect of alleviating pain using various forms of exercise. Specifically, it shows that in those with a directional preference who centralize, it does matter what exercises are prescribed and that guideline-based care is very much inferior to the use of exercises that match the directional preference identified at baseline. Further, this was true whether the patient's pain was acute or chronic, and whether they were having LBP-only or sciatica with a mild neurological deficit.

Additional discussion points regarding the Long study

Is two weeks sufficient follow-up for measuring efficacy? The issue of long term effects of treatment is an important one, but this was not ethically possible to study within the Long et al design with so many drop-outs expected and then observed in two of the three treatment groups. However, given the support this study provides for the short-term treatment efficacy using exercises matching the baseline assessment findings, interest in evaluating the long term efficacy increases substantially.

But we must recognize that this study is about a pain relief intervention. Consequently, there is value in comparing it with studies of analgesic medications. The beneficial effect of the latter is measurable in just 3–4 hours and doesn't require even two weeks. So those focused on the need for long-term follow-up in the Long et al study are missing some important messages provided by these data. Of great importance, guideline-based care with neutral forms of exercising was *interfering with* improvement, as measured by every other outcome measure, in more than half the subjects. It even caused 15% of those subjects, who otherwise would be expected to have a good outcome, to worsen.

Meanwhile, 95% of the "matched" exercise group significantly lowered or eliminated their pain in just two weeks. That needs to be said again: 95% of the "matched" exercise group significantly lowered or even eliminated their pain in just two weeks. Has there ever been any LBP intervention that effective? These patients spanned all duration categories (acute, subacute and chronic) and also LBP-only and sciatica subjects, yet they were all homogenous in that each had a directional preference and centralized identified at baseline.

It is rare that an RCT collects outcome measures as early as two weeks after the start of treatment. One of the benefits of doing so is to document just how early and quickly LBP and leg pain can be controlled and eliminated using directional preference-specific exercises. Both extensive clinical experience and published evidence report that centralization and directional preference are very often elicited on the day of initial assessment.[30, 31, 51, 52, 64, 75, 76, 116, 158, 161] It is in fact very common for patients to eliminate their own pain in just two or three days, or within one week. Most do not need the whole two weeks allowed in this study design.

Thus one question in need of future study: just how quickly does improvement with matching directional exercises occur? Waiting to begin the collection of outcomes until two weeks may not be a sufficiently short time span to capture the rapidity with which directional preference exercises can centralize, abolish, and then begin to prevent the return of pain. Waiting for six or twelve weeks to collect the first follow-up data, a much more common follow-up pattern, has no chance of capturing such rapid recoveries.

This study's generalizability. The Long et al study excluded only 23% of the consecutive LBP patients presenting for care. These percentages make the study much more generalizable than most. With the resulting study group including acute, subacute, and chronic, as well as LBP-only and sciatica, and with a 95% improvement rate with MDT treatment, it obviously makes little difference the duration of symptoms or whether the pain is local in the low back or all the way down the leg. Patients in whom a directional preference is elicited at baseline do very well if treated with directional preference–specific care (McKenzie/MDT).

Are guideline recommendations safe to use? Given that the MDT assessment had uncovered a directional preference in every patient included in this study, it is not surprising that some patients (15%) said they were worsened by exercises that took them in the direction opposite their directional preference.[90] This is of no great consequence given that no clinicians to my knowledge advocate treating LBP with such an exercise strategy.

What should be of some concern is the safety of patients treated with evidence-based care since 15% of this large directional preference subgroup so treated reported they worsened. But this form of care follows the recommendations of most recent guidelines. Therefore these data must be carefully considered. Further, one prominent systematic review concluded that general exercise may be beneficial for chronic LBP but there was no evidence back in 2000 that any specific exercise was any more effective than another.[144] That conclusion must now be reconsidered in light of these four subgroup specific RCTs that report a specific type of exercise as better than either alternative types or better than evidence-based care.[17, 18, 90, 121] Guideline groups must also reconsider and then revise their recommendations in light of this new evidence that, in the directional preference subgroup in particular, there are efficacious subgroup-specific exercises—with evidence of some risk of worsening if treatment followed currently recommended care.

Sciatica with directional preference. This centralization/directional preference subgroup embraces patients not usually included in the non-specific-LBP subgroup, namely those with sciatica and neurological deficits related to herniated discs. One cohort study focused entirely on patients with sciatica, once again reporting that centralizers, even with sciatica, had much better non-operative outcomes than non-centralizers.[129] Thus this large centralization/directional preference subgroup is not confined to those with non-specific LBP but also includes at least 50% of those with sciatica and neurological loss.[5, 80, 129]

Convention has placed LBP-only patients into the non-specific-LBP black box and sciatica into a distinctly different box. That must be re-thought however in light of these studies showing that most LBP-only and perhaps half of the sciatica subset have something very important in common: large percentages with a rapidly reversible pathology based on having a directional preference, often evident by eliciting the centralization response.

The implications of this are quite important. What does this say regarding a similarity in the anatomic and mechanical source of pain for LBP-only and those with sciatica? Most clinicians and researchers recognize the validity of disc pathology as the source of sciatica but we now must rethink whether the disc may be the underlying pain source for all those with LBP-only who have a directional preference. Again, the prevalence data for that subgroup for those with acute LBP is 70% or more. We'll return to this important topic in Chapter 10.

Correcting the underlying pathology: the basis for recovery of all outcome measures? What also seems clear from the Long et al study is that, not only were these directional exercises effective in reducing and eliminating pain, but every other outcome measure (depression, medication use, activity interference, and function) was substantially improved as well. In other words, teaching someone how to use an intervention that directly addresses their pain-generating disorder also produces the secondary benefits of improving one's functional abilities, one's depression, and stopping or decreasing medication use.

If all those issues occurred as a result of the onset and persistence of their LBP, wouldn't we expect that those same secondary issues would either improve or resolve if we have effectively dealt with the underlying problem? This is in substantial contrast to the psychosocial literature that postulates that patients with disability in time discover a type of "upside" to their condition, that is, they have less responsibilities and gain more attention because of their needs. Many therefore think that resolving chronic LBP is therefore more complex, and in some cases, this is certainly true. However, in the Long et al study, depression and chronic pain, along with any other unmeasured psychosocial characteristics obviously turned out to be non-obstacles to their rapid improvement or recovery in just two weeks for this large directional preference subgroup.

MDT clinicians' extensive experience has been: "Resolve the pain and the psychological manifestations resolve as well." Some very enlightening research can be done in this area.

There is also a very relevant systematic review to consider here that included trials of therapeutic exercises for LBP where a baseline effort was made to classify subjects using patient response methods.[32] Four out of five qualified studies reported improvement when the outcomes of a specific exercise program determined by the baseline symptom response were compared to those of a control group. The centralization pain response and McKenzie methods were common features of all the studies and the trials included patients who ranged from acute to chronic LBP. The review concluded that the patient response method of classification demonstrates a positive trend toward improving the likelihood of targeting the correct supervised exercises for patient intervention.

I mentioned that there have been four RCTs that have looked specifically at centralization and directional preference. The third is yet to be published but was presented at a recent international spine conference.[18] It randomized patients with symptoms distal to the buttock that centralized or abolished with extension during baseline evaluation. A full MDT evaluation was not provided, unfortunately, but it utilized the Delitto assessment process that tested only extension with repeated end-range movements, and the exam was conducted by those with little if any formal McKenzie Institute training. Their centralization prevalence has yet to be reported in this sample, although this research group had previously reported only a thirty percent prevalence.[63] Nevertheless, beginning at one-week and persisting through the six-month follow-up, the extension exercise treatment produced significantly better Oswestry Disability Questionnaire outcomes than did a lumbar stabilization exercise program. The authors concluded that directional preference and centralization were important sub-grouping criteria.

The fourth RCT also used the Delitto evaluation methods of sub-grouping. This classification system identifies three major subgroups, one of which is characterized as centralizers with a directional preference. Members of this subgroup are then treated with exercises in the matching direction. A 2006 RCT targeting all three of their major categories showed that outcomes when treatments were matched to patients' baseline subgroups were superior to using non-matching treatments.[17] The authors concluded that non-specific LBP was not a homogenous condition and that, just as we have seen in the Long study, outcomes can be significantly improved when subgroups are determined and then used to guide treatment decision-making.

I should also mention an earlier RCT that focused on McKenzie care but it was a black box RCT in that it studied acute patients with non-specific LBP.[25] It randomized these patients to MDT by Credentialed physical therapists as one of three interventions. Consequently, the McKenzie assessment took place after randomization and, unfortunately, no subgroup data was collected to enable an analysis of the centralizing and directional preference subgroup. Furthermore, the McKenzie arm was not permitted to exclude patients for whom the MDT assessment indicated would be unresponsive to MDT treatment

Nevertheless, one might have expected there to be a large extension directional preference subgroup whose excellent outcomes would dominate the results and give an advantage to McKenzie care. Such was not the case. While McKenzie care showed trends toward being more efficacious, and while it certainly matched the efficacy of chiropractic care as one of the other treatment arms in the study, there were no statistically significant differences between the outcomes for McKenzie care, chiropractic care or an educational booklet.

<u>Does it matter which exercise is prescribed?</u> Incredibly, it is rarely acknowledged in the LBP exercise research that there are different forms of exercise with different intents. The purpose and role of these directional exercises is clear and unique. They are not for strengthening, stretching or conditioning. Their intent is very specific: to apply beneficial loads to the pain-generating pathology in such a way that the low back and leg symptoms produced by that pathology centralize and abolish and are then prevented from returning. In the properly selected patients, they appear to correct a rapidly reversible spinal pathology.

Three of these RCTs compared the effects of two different forms of exercise in acute LBP patients, especially those found to have a directional preference. The results of all three studies showed a significant difference in outcomes between various forms of exercise. These three should then significantly alter the conclusions of the next systematic review of exercise therapy for acute LBP. Indeed, one of the main conclusions of the last substantial exercise systematic review was the absence of evidence that specific exercises were effective for the treatment of acute low back pain.[144]

All these studies have the same message: sub-group classification of LBP seems to be the most promising in terms of getting beyond the trivial treatment effects and minimal differences to which we've grown accustomed from black box RCTs.

Summary

Although more RCTs are needed to corroborate the results of these four studies, the consistency of findings of these four, in combination with all the outcome predictive cohort studies,[56, 65, 72, 88, 90, 129, 136, 157, 158] is quite impressive.

What is equally impressive to me and to the thousands of MDT-trained clinicians around the world, all these study results are precisely what is daily seen in thousands of clinical practices everyday, in the U.S., Canada, New Zealand, Australia, across all of Europe, Brazil, India, Kuwait, Russia, China, Japan, South Africa, Nigeria and a host of other countries. This vast clinical network reports that most LBP patients around the world are centralizers with a directional preference who achieve swift pain and functional recovery using patient-specific directional exercises and compatible posture modifications. And these results are seen clinically in acutes and chronics, and in LBP-only and sciatica, just as these data report. Unfortunately, non-MDT clinicians and all other LBP stakeholders do not have the benefit of this internal validity.

Given the strength of the current validation for, and the sheer size of, the centralization/directional preference subgroup, designing studies over the next ten years to learn more about this subgroup and its many repercussions and implications will no doubt provide the research goldmine to which we referred earlier in terms of substantially increasing our understanding of the mechanisms and management of LBP. We'll examine that goldmine further in Chapter 10.

Meanwhile, Spratt's A–D–T–O research model is such a simple, coherent guide for interpreting existing and planning future studies that, if implemented, will greatly diminish the use of black box RCTs that have so dominated the LBP literature and have actually become obstacles to our progress in understanding LBP.

Chapter 9

Implications of Rapidly Reversible Low Back Pain

To be effective, treatment must somehow reach and reverse the painful process at its source in a lasting fashion. If one is not successful reversing the pain-generating disorder, it will persist, allowing pre-existing psychosocial factors to become operative, flourish, and even dominate.

—James Cyriax, MD

Obstacles to recovery: old and new

Clinical LBP research has been focused heavily on the chronic population largely because such a high percentage of LBP costs are spent on this group. Given the conventional view that acute LBP is a benign disorder (see discussion in Chapter 4), it makes good economic sense to attempt to identify factors that might prevent recovery and cause acute LBP to become chronic.

Consequently, over the past two decades, a great deal of research has focused on identifying and analyzing what are now commonly referred to as "obstacles to recovery." A prominent trend in this research is the focus on certain psychosocial factors; i.e., the so-called "yellow flags" that can play a role in prolonging LBP and disability. We will discuss this psychosocial topic in some detail later in this chapter.

However published data report that the pain of 50% of chronics can be centralized and abolished and they can still achieve a good prognosis.[80, 88-90] Given that so many respond so well and even recover with Mechanical Diagnosis and Therapy (MDT) even after their problem becomes chronic, the question arises as to why these folks don't recover much earlier, either on their own or with some other form of treatment?

It is important to understand that *when the MDT assessment of an individual with chronic LBP reveals them to be a centralizer with a directional preference, their underlying pain generator no doubt possessed that rapidly reversible characteristic from the time they were acute.* That is not a feature that their pain generator acquired after they became chronic. It was there all the time but was simply undiscovered, for months, some-times even for years. This persistent rapid reversibility characteristic was simply never detected because the care provider(s) either never considered it or perhaps didn't realize such a turn-around could even occur and therefore never looked for it. But once these patients are finally provided an opportunity to be examined in this way and centralization and directional preference are elicited, most of these chronic patients have very good outcomes when treated appropriately.

But what has been these chronic centralizers' obstacle to recovery all this time that was then apparently addressed? That question is more easily answered by considering the nature of the intervention responsible for the rather abrupt recovery. Since the successful intervention was essentially mechanical and relatively rapid in bringing about recovery, it is unlikely that any behavioral issues identified at baseline were major obstacles to recovery, as is so commonly considered in these chronic patients. Even more convincing are the data supporting that a successful MDT intervention can overcome and even reverse documented baseline psychosocial issues such as depression, fear avoidance, and perceived disability.[90, 157] As we stated in Chapter 8, the experience of most MDT clinicians is: "resolve the pain and the psychological manifestations resolve as well."

For this centralizing and directional preference subgroup that may comprise as much as 50% of chronic patients, it is clear that the only obstacle to their recovery was their care provider(s) not providing this specific form of MDT assessment. That obstacle is unfortunately too common across all disciplines in low back care.

Once these chronic patients see how easily and simply they can centralize, eliminate and even prevent their chronic pain, two very common patient responses are: "I can't believe it's this easy," and "Why didn't someone show me this long, long ago?" illustrating this huge obstacle to low back pain recovery. Though this is a clinician-related obstacle, the good news is that it can be remedied with effective physi-cian education tied to guideline revisions acknowledging that the lack of an MDT assessment can be a potential obstacle to recovery.

One of my objectives in writing this book is to bring attention to this obstacle so LBP patients might not be deprived of this opportunity to recover while also sparing payers the high costs of so many unnecessary and expensive diagnostic and treatment interventions.

Is MDT for everyone with LBP?

To answer this question requires making a very important distinction between MDT assessment and treatment. This distinction is unclear to those who think MDT is treatment only, and that it more specifically equates to the use of extension exercises only. It is truly remarkable how many LBP experts have no appreciation for the MDT assessment, especially considering that McKenzie's original text has been widely available for 25 years along with hundreds of McKenzie educational courses taught around the world and many published review articles during that same time.

But please realize that the *MDT assessment is for everyone with LBP.* To best illustrate, let's consider some extreme examples. In the case of an undiagnosed fracture, tumor, or some other red flag, MDT *treatment* is quite inappropriate yet MDT *assessment* would neither be contraindicated or inappropriate. To the contrary, my experience is that the MDT clinician is much more likely to make or suspect such a diagnosis based on the findings of their thorough methods of history taking and the MDT spinal testing simply because the pain patterns of these insidious LBP sources are so very distinct from the patterns related to the three McKenzie syndromes: derangement, dysfunction or posture. With the MDT exam being so safe because these pain patterns are so closely monitored throughout, the unique pain patterns of red flag pathologies are quickly, clearly, and safely exposed so these patients can be promptly moved on to more extensive and focused assessment of their serious underlying pathology. Physicians who refer their patients for MDT assessment are always grateful to have such a thorough means of assessment backing them up should they have missed such a diagnosis with their own history and exam.

Although there are no published data as yet about the MDT exam findings of such patients, there are many remarkable anecdotal stories of referrals for MDT evaluation for what the referring physician felt was mechanical LBP, only to have the MDT assessment promptly determine that this pain and its underlying source were clearly not mechanical and in need of further evaluation. With such rapid feedback from the MDT clinician, the referring physician can then re-evaluate and move the patient toward a more focused red flag evaluation.

There are also the irreducible derangements, those whose pain does not centralize, indeed it seems to worsen with all directions of test movement. These patients will not respond to MDT treatment and are in need of further diagnostic and treatment interventions. They are either patients with sciatica[80] or have an internal disc disruption that can be demonstrated with discography.[50, 82] MRI or CT imaging and epidural injections are commonly considered and, of course, some even require surgery. The MDT assessment process is extremely informative in this subgroup even though MDT treatment is of little benefit.

We also discussed the "Other" subgroup in Chapter 7. This comprises only a small percentage of the acute patient population but fortunately, and importantly, these patients can be identified early so time and expense is not wasted on unproductive care. This group is among the non-centralizers that have a poor prognosis at one-year follow-up[157] but, to date, there has been very little research focused on this small subgroup.

Thus, MDT *assessment* can indeed be for everyone with LBP and I'd personally recommend it for everyone, assuming it is accessible. Essentially all my own patients underwent this form of assessment by a well-trained MDT clinician as part of their initial evaluation with me. In the eyes of a growing number of LBP clinicians, the assessment's potential to provide so much important information at so little cost and with little, if any, risk provides too much value to neglect its routine inclusion in the baseline assessment process.

So MDT *assessment* is for everyone while MDT *treatment* is appropriate for 70+% of acute patients who are centralizers plus those who fit MDT's dysfunction and posture syndromes.

Natural history revisited

While we discussed the natural history of LBP at some length in Chapter 4, it is worth revisiting in light of what we are learning about so many patients' pain response patterns and directional themes.

You'll recall that we reviewed several population studies [34, 145, 146, 152, 153] that report that the natural history of LBP is not as favorable as is claimed in past and current guidelines. A high percentage (69–82%) of LBP sufferers are still having symptoms one year after onset and 25% are still having substantial limitation to their activities. That's quite a contrast to the recent guideline natural history description stating that "recovery occurs in 90% within 6 weeks with only 2%–7% developing chronic pain."[143] The term "recovery" of course needs a uniform definition, but when high percentages of both persisting symptoms and activity restriction persist at one year, few would qualify those people as fully "recovered."

Despite these data however, the natural history of LBP remains generally favorable. Recovery with no formal care is still common, especially amongst those who never seek care, even though the LBP may return as recurrent episodes. However, the recovery rate through natural history is probably nowhere near as high as it is routinely reported in guidelines.

So why is recovery as favorable as it is? Is it merely due to the passage of time?

Recovery by natural history

Although there has been so much attention given to identifying obstacles to recovery, one completely overlooked topic and I think an important key to improving our understanding of LBP is to consider and investigate *how people do recover*. Rather than studying the non-recovering population, why is it that so many recover from their LBP episodes? And can the literature we've reviewed regarding pain patterns and directional preference offer any new insights into those recoveries that occur without formal treatment? Is LBP recovery simply based on the "tincture of time," as a condition that just has to run its course, like the common cold?

Let's begin by considering the high percentage (~70%) who experience recurrences. For them, the recurrent nature of their LBP is at the heart of their low back problem. For them, it's a part of their LBP natural history, perhaps "natural history-part 2."

When you think about it, recurrences represent both good and bad news. The bad news of course is that the episodes keep recurring and, in many cases, as we also discussed in Chapter 4, even progressively worsen. On the other hand, the good news is that these episodes keep recovering. It's that recurrent pattern of pain, first coming and then going, that seems to further reflect the very common *reversible* character of the underlying pain source. Do you notice how this "reversible LBP" term and concept keeps popping up?

Meanwhile, the ability to improve recovery rates with evidence-based care has been documented now in several studies. Altering the population's understanding of LBP within one Australian state through public service education about its benign nature and the benefits of remaining active significantly reduced disability and workers' compensation costs compared with no such education in another control state.[19] Another Australian study utilized a case-control patient audit design that showed marginally better short-term and significantly better long-term results when evidence-based care was introduced in special clinics compared to the usual acute low back care provided by general practitioners.[99, 100]

So there seems to be some benefit in orienting low back treatment around the one-size-fits-all guideline approach of encouraging people to remain active. But why is that? Why does LBP recover more frequently by having people remain more active?

Reversible LBP

Does the term "reversible LBP" characterize recurrent episodes just as it does the directional pain responses elicited within the MDT assessment process? Does this very common LBP reversibility reflect a characteristic of a common type of LBP-generator that is revealed in a variety of pain monitoring circumstances? What seems apparent is that one set of circumstances, likely mechanical in most cases, "turns on" or starts an episode and then some other set of circumstances allows it to turn off again. For those with many episodes, that cycle obviously repeats itself over and over.

But what turns the pain on and off? When people recover "on their own" for example, is it merely the passage of time or do some other circumstances provide their pain source with something beneficial that enables recovery? If some set of circumstances enables recovery in some, are there dissimilar circumstances that somehow prevent recovery in another?

What do guideline recommendations mean by "remain active"?

Stay with me on this now. Clinical guidelines recommend that clinicians encourage LBP patients to remain active. That sounds straightforward enough ... at first. Ironically, no guidance has ever been provided as to just what "remain active" means in guidelines. So is just any activity good? Or are there some activities that are not particularly good, perhaps even bad, that might even serve as obstacles to recovery?

Whereas LBP clinicians are instructed to encourage activity, how many of them would actually recommend that their LBP patients resume their work in the garden, vacuuming, mopping, shoveling snow, lifting, or bending repeatedly? After all, these all represent different forms of remaining active.

Although guidelines strongly recommend keeping LBP patients active, they are in fact silent regarding any specifics. Ironically, this is in great contrast to most physicians who have very clear opinions on this point.

I earlier mentioned the survey of all 38 general practitioners attending a general medical conference. They were also queried about any "activity instructions" they give their LBP patients.[54] It was quite revealing as they were unanimous on three specific things. Every one of them instructed their patients to: 1) pursue walking, 2) avoid lifting, and 3) avoid sitting in a slouched position. Further, 75% said they also instructed their LBP patients to avoid forward bending and sit-ups but instructed them to always sit erectly.

Does that sound like these docs recognize that lumbar flexion is a bad thing to do and should be avoided? And consider this: walking is the single activity we all perform on a regular basis that does not bend our lumbar spines in a forward direction. In fact, compared with our otherwise flexed or forward-bent lifestyle, walking is "relative extension" for the lumbar spine.

Does that resemble a directional preference for extension? They are clearly saying to their patients: avoid flexion and remain erect by either walking or sitting up tall; that is, in relative extension.

But where did they acquire this notion of giving directional activity instructions to their LBP patients? And why is this notion so universally held? After all, most physicians haven't read about directional preference in the scientific literature and they certainly didn't get this from reading LBP clinical guidelines.

Some assistance is provided by the survey of 349 LBP care-seekers seeing general practitioners, surgeons, chiropractors and physical therapists. One portion of the survey focused on how patients said their LBP responded to seventeen common movements, positions, and activities, each of which would require either some form of lumbar flexion (forward bending) or being upright.[54] Of the nine flexion items, *every one* was graded by the surveyed patients as more aggravating to their pain than the eight upright items that were all graded as more comfortable (p<0.0001).

I would submit that the activity instructions so commonly provided by physicians to avoid flexion and remain erect have been described to them over and over by their patients. Clinicians perhaps gain this insight via something akin to osmosis: a constant bombardment of information that eventually seeps into the mind. Another credible explanation is that most LBP clinicians have likely experienced LBP of their own, coming to realize that some things reduced their pain (like being erect) while others (like bending, lifting, sneezing) caused or increased their pain, sometimes even to a remarkably strong pain experience.

So how do people recover on their own?

While it is obviously unnecessary to know the pain source to recover from LBP, one human characteristic may hold the key to recovery. Benjamin Franklin put it this way: "We are first moved by pain, and the whole succeeding course of our lives is but one continuous series of actions with a view to be freed from it."

Isn't that how most LBP sufferers respond to things that increase their pain? They instinctively try to avoid them, except in cases where there is some other overbearing reason to perform the activity and endure the pain. Even without their doctor's instructions, and despite guidelines' silence on what activities to avoid, our own backs quickly teach us that bending, lifting, and prolonged slouched sitting aggravates our problem. So we of course avoid, or try to minimize, those activities and positions that aggravate pain, thus reducing the mechanical aggravation of our back disorder that in turn provides the pain source with a greater opportunity for recovery.

In essence, encouraging patients to remain active promotes activity that requires painful backs to move and change positions that in turn reveals to patients what their painful backs like and don't like. By monitoring their own pain, the natural thing for anyone to do, many patients learn quickly that their backs tolerate erect walking and sitting so much better than they do bending or slouched sitting. They then temporarily modify their day by walking more and sitting and bending much less. So just as in the MDT assessment, they learn from their pain the same directional theme that every one of the surveyed doctors also recognized: the value of being erect and the hazards of sitting, bending, and lifting. So left to themselves, patients seem to perform their own version of an MDT assessment, minus the specific repetitive end-range testing in multiple directions that so often adds so much information about the pain source to further guide their recovery strategy.

There is also ample documentation that it is flexed positions that so often bring on LBP,[91] and flexion that also aggravates the pain once started.[52, 55, 81, 90, 131, 135, 160] But it is being erect, either walking or supported sitting (relative lumbar extension), that so often feels much better.[55, 131, 160]

Thus, if the directional pattern of low back-related symptoms truly reflects a directional characteristic of the underlying pain-generator, then one would expect to find internal validity for these directional themes emerging from patients' pain response to both daily activities and the spinal testing as part of the MDT assessment.

Consequently, it appears the favorable natural history of LBP may in many cases be related to recovery of a reversible pain generator with a directional preference that responds favorably to a directional self-care strategy determined by patients themselves as they attempt to avoid painful lumbar flexion and pursue more erect sitting and walking.

Then why does LBP so often persist?

Hippocrates said: "Healing is a matter of time, but it is also a matter of opportunity." How true. Providing directional self-care to a pain source with a directional preference may well be providing that pain source with the opportunity to recover.

So despite the fact that healing does take time, judicious use of that time is required to provide the opportunity for recovery. A simple cut needs time to heal, but it also needs the opportunity and favorable circumstances, perhaps with stitches, or at least a protective bandage and some disinfectant. Alternatively, the very same time spent pulling the cut apart, scratching or tearing at it, or getting it dirty, will greatly prolong, or prevent healing altogether. Such persisting trauma or aggravation can even create a far worse problem than the original cut. So while time is certainly necessary for healing, time spent without the provision of opportunity is insufficient. It is the combination of time and opportunity that enables healing to occur.

So what happens when pain persists, even to the point of becoming chronic? First of all, it is somewhat astonishing to me when low back experts state or write that most acute LBP would usually recover and heal within six weeks, as though time alone is sufficient. What often then follows are statements that pain that lasts longer than three months is likely not from the original physical injury that would and should have healed in that time. To explain the persisting pain, it is then hypothesized that persisting chronic LBP must therefore be due to some other mechanism that gets "turned on" in certain people, such as some version of psychosocial somatization or the activation or augmentation of a central pain processing mechanism within the dorsal horns of the spinal cord.[104, 137]

While these latter explanations may be credible for some individuals, it also seems that the simple and wider recognition of the persistence of a physical pain source from repeated irritation of the original physical pain generator has far greater probability of occurring here, but is never acknowledged as a possible mechanism for persisting pain.

When was the last time you heard or read that chronic low back symptoms could be related to the original physical injury? This is not only conceivable, it could obviously occur quite commonly if the pain source undergoes repeated physical insults that prevent its healing so it evolves into a worse condition than when it started. Just like the skin cut, for LBP to recover and remain so, sufferers must somehow provide their underlying disorder with both the opportunity and the time it needs to recover. But if either the cut or one's low back disorder is frequently aggravated, the pain is sure to persist independent of the presence or absence of any psychosocial factors.

The biopsychosocial model: what is it and how does rapidly reversible LBP relate to it?

The biopsychosocial model for thinking about chronic LBP has emerged over the past 25 years to a place of prominence. It is commonly tied to discussions of why LBP becomes chronic in some individuals and not others. What prevents certain individuals from recovering?

In combination with the lack of a "valid" diagnosis in the eyes of many for the majority with LBP, a substantial body of psychosocial research has evolved to the point where behavioral factors have become a mainstay in current LBP guidelines.

The early phase of the biopsychosocial model

The biopsychosocial model emerged in the '80s largely in response to the failure of medicine to identify good biological causes and treatments for LBP coupled with a growing sense that LBP was being "over-medicalized." This latter consideration was especially focused on the many in whom some anatomic target for surgical intervention was allegedly found that then required one or more surgeries, unfortunately with many unsuccessful outcomes.

The patient's perception of their own LBP came to be viewed as highly influenced by social and psychological factors, including one's emotional response to illness, that is their illness behavior.[59, 87] A progressive shift in thinking then took place toward a greater appreciation for the relevance of these psychosocial factors in acute LBP becoming chronic.[149, 150] The acceptance of this model grew as a credible construct in which to introduce, expand on, and view the role of psychosocial factors in individuals' LBP experience.

More recent interpretation of the biopsychosocial model in LBP

Over the past 20 years, this psychosocial domain has played an increasingly prominent role in how LBP is viewed by primary care researchers, especially how LBP so often becomes chronic. Studies and theories have led to the conceptualization of so-called *yellow flags*, intended to represent risk factors or potential obstacles to recovery, and therefore factors in need of attention, in an attempt to avoid chronicity.

Coupled with our inability to identify a physical cause of LBP in 85% of patients, it is not surprising that many patients with persisting or chronic non-specific LBP report the presence of psychosocial issues. Some of these factors, like depression and fear-avoidance are documented to be present at baseline in many with acute LBP. Although the biopsychosocial pendulum was for many years positioned at the "bio" end of the biopsychosocial continuum when "over-medicalizing" was so prominent, the psychosocial research of the '80s and '90s has led consensus guidelines to swing that pendulum strongly away from the "bio" end and toward the opposite psychosocial end of the continuum as one now views chronic LBP (see Figure 9–1).

Has the biopsychosocial pendulum now swung too far toward the psychosocial end?

Many have entered the field of LBP research during and since the '90s who have been strongly influenced by the past 10–15 years of psychosocial research in which such factors have been widely viewed as common contributors to LBP becoming chronic. I think a broader perspective on this whole biopsychosocial topic however is helpful.

A common line of thought is that, if there was a physical cause or causes for LBP, our high levels of technology and knowledge would have identified it. In other words, the "absence of proof" of an anatomic cause has been commonly and illogically interpreted as the "proof of absence" of a physical source of LBP. We talked a bit about this in our previous section. The belief by some that we have exhausted all possibilities for identifying physical causes has caused concern amongst some researchers and clinicians that the psychosocial view of chronic LBP is excessively applied.

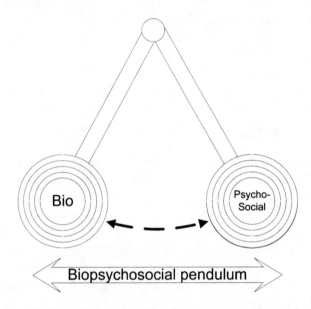

Figure 9–1: The biopsychosocial pendulum has swung in recent years from what many feel was an over-medicalization extreme (far left) to what many now feel is an over-psychosocializing extreme in the opposite direction (far right).

Historically, when the biopsychosocial pendulum was first conceptualized, it helped swing it away from the "bio" end to escape what was perceived as over-medicalizing. However, it has just kept swinging in that same direction to where, according to most guidelines, it should now reside. But some, including myself, are just as concerned about characterizing all of chronic LBP as predominantly psychosocial. We may be repeating a similar pattern of extremism by now "over-psycho-socializing" chronic LBP just as we once "over-medicalized" it.

Do we really have a "proof of absence" of a physical cause? Are biologic sources of LBP assumed to be absent just because of our deficiencies in detecting them? Does the presence of psychosocial factors at baseline provide a sufficient rationale for dismissing the presence of a physical cause to one's LBP? At the very least, we need to avoid assuming there is no longer a physical source and remain open to finding new ways to identify these sources.

Is rapid reversibility a pathway to recovery and cost savings?

The biopsychosocial model of back pain is a useful model for understanding the whole of the LBP population; that is, until one tries to characterize all of chronic LBP as lying at one specific point along that continuum. In my view, this is a trap set by focusing only on aggregated or group mean differences from black box RCTs. Remember and consider that within that chronic population, A–D–T–O data (see Chapter 8) indicate that many individuals, perhaps as high as 50%, have a reversible, biologic source of pain (the centralization/directional preference subgroup) while another important subgroup has very operative psychosocial factors in need of cognitive-behavioral care. And then there are some with both, in whom the initial focus should always be on treating the physical since the behavioral issues so often become inactive when the pain is effectively addressed.[90, 157]

Again, the many centralization studies provide strong evidence that a large chronic LBP subgroup has possessed for the entire time they've been symptomatic, an undetected, reversible physical disorder as their primary source of pain. Some of these folks might also have identifiable psychosocial factors that, either in the absence of, or in the case of undetected centralization/directional preference, could become obstacles to their recovery. At least one high-quality prospective outcome study of acute LBP reported that baseline psychosocial factors became inactive as predictors of chronicity in the large subgroup of acute patients who also exhibited a centralization pain pattern at baseline.[157] *Undetected* centralization/directional preference, being as common as it is, may well be a far more common obstacle to recovery than are psychosocial factors.

Despite these MDT methodologies being well-described for the past 25 years, and with extensive published research over the past 15 years, it is ironic and unfortunate that so many LBP clinicians and researchers are unaware of the value provided by searching for these pain patterns. And nowhere have the unintended consequences of black box RCTs been more apparent than in guideline generalizations that chronic LBP is so heavily influenced by psychosocial issues, a conclusion justified by black box statistical means, with no regard for subgrouping. In considering the huge prevalence of LBP and the personal and societal expense of the problem, it would seem there is a great need to identify valid LBP subgroups using the A–D–T–O model for research strategy.

The key therefore to applying the biopsychosocial model clinically is to identify ways to more objectively evaluate each individual, rather than generalizing about their condition based on one's view of the biopsychosocial pendulum swing. The question of whether we are over-medicalizing or over-psychosocializing chronic LBP becomes moot if we have the means to objectively determine where each individual might fall along that continuum. What may appear an appropriate generalization for a group as a whole will often be inappropriate for any individual. We must treat individuals, not statistical means, and by treating individuals with patient-specific care, the costs of care will no doubt drop substantially.

At the end of the day, the prevailing question for every clinician, as well as for every clinical researcher, remains: how do we make decisions regarding individuals in the exam room? Where does this patient fit along the continuum of the biopsychosocial model? It is inappropriate to address a patient based on statistical means and the conclusions of systematic reviews or guidelines. Does he or she have an identifiable physical cause, or perhaps some relevant psychosocial issue(s), or both?

On one hand, we know that *the onset* of LBP is rarely related to a person's psychosocial profile but is typically physical and predominantly mechanical. We also know that depression is more often a consequence of unresolved LBP than is LBP a consequence of depression. Even those with prior psychosocial issues are hardly immune to the onset of LBP from mechanical origin. Obviously, depression can also have many other causes than LBP.

As we know, the identification and treatment of a physical pain source, whether it is back or abdominal pain, clearly takes precedent. In that context, searching for, and then treating centralization/directional preference should be the priority, regardless of a patient's psychosocial profile.[90] Documented baseline psychosocial factors in acute LBP patients have been shown to become non-issues and non-predictors of outcome in patients in whom centralization was found and directly addressed.[157] On the other hand, in those found in that same study to be non-centralizers, there was also a strong prediction of a poor behavioral response (coping) to spine pain. Specifically, members of the small

> "The key therefore to applying the biopsychosocial model clinically is to identify ways to more objectively evaluate each individual, rather than generalizing about their condition based on one's view of the biopsychosocial pendulum swing."

non-centralizing subgroup, compared with centralizers, were nine times more likely to have non-organic signs, thirteen times more likely to have overt pain behaviors, three times more likely to have fear of work, and two times more likely to have somatization.[156]

A strong word of caution is in order here however. These data by no means indicate that all or even most non-centralizers have these behavioral issues and characteristics. For example, if centralizers only demonstrated psychosocial factors 2% of the time, then non-organic signs would have only been present in 18% of non-centralizers.

Alternative views of why pain complaints so often persist

This pendulum swing to the psychosocial end of the spectrum does not, in the view of many, adequately explain the persistence of chronic pain complaints. Could there be other mechanisms perpetuating symptoms that originally arose from some physical low back problem that would or should have recovered within a few weeks or months, at least hypothetically? After all, many say "we *know* the original cause of the pain has recovered and can no longer be a pain source." Do we? We discussed the flaws in this assumption earlier in this chapter.

Consequently, a completely new basic science research focus has unfolded in an attempt to explain the persistence of LBP in many chronics. Various forms of spinal cord activation and excitability are being identified that are presumed to be perpetuating and facilitating pain messages traveling to the brain long after the original spinal pain source has allegedly recovered or healed.[104, 137] Advanced brain imaging of pain perception is another fascinating area of research trying to explain chronic pain perception.

So the chronic LBP population is currently perceived by many low back experts, and especially amongst low back primary care researchers, as dominated by psychosocial factors and central nervous system pain-generating and perception mechanisms that become activated as chronic sources of perceived LBP.

But what about the 50% of chronics that demonstrate centralization and directional preference and therefore have such a good prognosis for recovery? Are we not compelled to look at this subset of chronic pain from a very different perspective?[50, 82, 88, 90]

The cognitive-behavioral element of MDT

No physical treatment or patient-provider interaction is void of behavioral influences on patients. No doubt the cognitive-behavioral benefits of MDT are likely substantial, and this represents another fascinating and untapped area for future research.

Within MDT, many cognitive domains can be involved. As patients learn the usefulness of their pain response patterns elicited during their assessments, they learn, not how to cope with their pain, but how to gain control over it and then eliminate it. Such empowerment over their painful dilemma is powerful and a very satisfying accomplishment for both the patient and the treating clinician.

In keeping with current guideline recommendations, there is perhaps no stronger message of assurance of recovery than for patients to discover at the outset of their care that they can centralize and abolish their own pain. Although this first happens under the care and tutelage of the MDT clinician, patients routinely experience an even stronger sense of empowerment at home or at work when they are again able to eliminate any returning symptoms on their own using the same simple strategies they just learned in the clinic.

Transforming this clinical impression that a patient's rapid transition from having an external locus of control, where they feel victimized by their LBP, to an internal locus of control as they learn they can eliminate it into established empirical evidence is another research project waiting to happen. It is a means of documenting the beneficial psychosocial effect of quickly learning to control and eliminate their own symptoms. Such investigations will substantially contribute to the world's understanding of the interactions between the physical and psychosocial elements within individual patients.

Shrinking the black box

Let's briefly return to our Chapter 2 discussion of our current LBP clinical guidelines, which recommends that acute LBP be categorized using the "diagnostic triage," or what we have referred to in this book as the "black box" classification. Ironically, despite it being named "diagnostic" by so many experts, this model acknowledges that 85% of individuals with LBP have no identifiable diagnosis.

But now we have convincing data that 70% of individuals with acute LBP have a directional preference with centralizing pain and therefore also an excellent prognosis. Additionally, we have evidence that as many as 50% of patients with sciatica from a herniated disc (HD) also have a directional preference and, again, a very good prognosis. The remaining sciatica-HD patients are also classified as MDT derangements, but they are irreducible or irreversible and part of the non-centralizing subgroup.

This all means that the MDT derangements, including the directional preference/centralization subgroup in particular, comprise a very high percentage of patients who would otherwise have landed in the non-specific-LBP black box. This includes many within the herniated disc category as well. When we subtract both reversible and irreversible derangements from the big black box of non-specific LBP (see Figure 2–2), this black box shrinks substantially from 85% of all LBP to perhaps less than 10% (see Figure 9–2). More precise data have not been gathered yet.

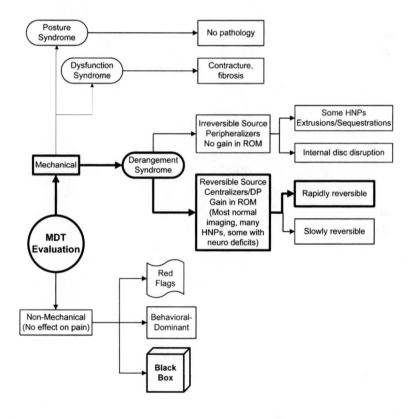

Figure 9–2: By identifying the very large rapidly reversible derangement subgroup, the "black box" of non-specific LBP is greatly reduced in size. Compare with Figure 2–2.

PART 4
The Benefits of Subgroup Identification

Chapter 10
Subgroups: A Goldmine for Managing and Understanding Low Back Pain

In most areas of medicine, identifying and validating patient subgroups is a major stepping stone that stimulates many new and fundamental questions about that subgroup. The value and importance of those questions increases directly with the size of the subgroup-of-interest.

Superimposed upon the abundance of directional preference validity evidence is data indicating the high prevalence of directional preference: over 70% of the acute and as high as 50% of the chronic LBP population. Consequently, interest in learning more about members of this very large subgroup should be very high on the part of all stakeholders, especially researchers.

At the 2004 International LBP Forum conference in Edmonton, Alberta, one discussant referred to the identification and investigation of LBP subgroups as "a gold mine," based on the many opportunities he envisioned to acquire new insights into back pain. As I thought about this comment, it occurred to me how much this resembled the Cochrane Back Review Group's reference to subgroup identification as "the Holy Grail" of LBP.[15] Validating subgroups will unlock so much of the LBP mystery. It does indeed resemble a LBP goldmine.

In the context of this large validated centralization/directional preference subgroup, there are so many extremely important areas of low back care and understanding that are worthy to consider and that need further investigation and should be of great interest to all LBP stakeholders:

1. the concept of rapid reversibility
2. clinical decision-making
3. predicting outcomes
4. understanding disease process
5. primary and secondary prevention
6. cost reduction
7. disease management low back care innovations
8. improving research design and interpretation

Let's take a brief look at each of these in light of the validation of this large directional preference subgroup.

Although most readers will find this next section ("The concept of rapid reversibility") worthwhile, some may find one or more of the subsequent topics in this chapter a bit too detailed or complex for their level of interest or understanding. If such is the case for you, skip ahead to those sections of greater interest. Note that the next chapter, Chapter 11, is especially relevant for researchers. Then Chapter 12 through the remainder of the book should have broader appeal again.

1. The concept of rapid reversibility

Let's first consider our current but meager *non*-MDT clinical examination skills or tools. Those shown to be reliable have pretty much been limited to the neurological exam, quantifying lumbar range-of-motion, and some pain provocative manual tests that have not yet been tied through the A–D–T–O model to any subgroup validity studies. Then also consider the substantial limitations of x-rays, CT, and MRI imaging in identifying with any confidence for non-red flag pain-generating sources. Then we have the difficulty that so many asymptomatic individuals have disc abnormalities, even herniations, on their images.[11, 12] Which discs with degenerative changes on MRI are symptomatic and which are not? We often simply do not know.

Discography is the only imaging study we have with any chance of tying disc morphology with symptoms. This form of imaging study is based on reproducing patients' exact or concordant pain simultaneously with an injection into the pain-generating disc. While it remains a controversial procedure in the eyes of many, it is still very informative when performed with properly selected patients.

Unfortunately, that covers the spectrum of the current mainstream evaluations for non-specific LBP or sciatica. But what is particularly absent is any form of exam that in any way tests and determines whether the underlying disorder is reversible or not, and if it is, is there any identifiable means of reversing it?

Consider this: although we don't use the word "reversible," clinicians are certainly encouraged by guideline recommendations to tell their acute LBP patients that they will likely get better in the next few weeks or so, regardless of which treatment they utilize. So it's not a matter of not knowing that most LBP is reversible, we know it usually is. But we also know that the problem often doesn't reverse on its own, as is the case with all those with symptoms that persist for months or years. But according to currently published data, 50% of chronic LBP patients are actually undetected centralizers; i.e., they have rapidly reversible pathology, but they just haven't been given the opportunity to undergo a reversibility evaluation.

So directional preference and centralization bring an entirely new layer of useful information to our understanding of LBP that we've never had before. If a patient's symptoms are reversible, the pathology they reflect must also be reversible and is usually also capable of remaining reversed (corrected, reduced) if the symptom reversal can be maintained, that is, keep the pain centralized and abolished. The extent to which this can be accomplished empowers patients to take and maintain control of, and then recover from, their conditions. Existing research following the A–D–T–O research model supports what MDT-trained clinicians have been claiming for years: their ability to inexpensively and safely test the pain-generator to determine whether it is or is not reversible.

No other diagnostic tool has ever provided such specific and valuable information about the pain-generating pathology. The MDT repeated movement exam, properly and thoroughly performed, is capable of providing a whole new dimension of information about the pain source: the "reversibility" of the underlying painful lesion.

If we return to McKenzie's term "derangement" to describe the type of mechanical pathology that seems evident in these patients (see Chapter 7), then a commonly used alternative to the term reversal of the pathology is "reduction," used to describe the re-locating of a displaced structure; i.e., reducing a shoulder dislocation or a displaced torn meniscus (commonly referred to as "internal derangements"). This term derangement captures the rapidity with which members of this large centralization/directional preference subgroup can eliminate their pain and restore their full range of motion. It is as though something displaced and painful has just been "reduced" or corrected.

Alternatively, there's a small subset of patients whose MDT exam findings indicate the presence of a derangement but their LBP and/ or radiating symptoms cannot be fully or sometimes even partially centralized or abolished. This subgroup's derangements are said to be "irreducible" or irreversible. We'll discuss this group further in the "Understanding Disease Process" section later in this chapter. They are depicted in Figure 9–2.

2. Clinical decision-making: who to treat, how to treat,

and who not to treat?

Let's suppose you are a clinician evaluating your new patient Sue who has come seeking your help with her LBP. Once you have ruled out the likelihood of any red flag pathologies causing her pain, one of your next priorities should be to classify Sue, if possible, into one of the three McKenzie syndromes, and especially to determine if she might be in that very large directional preference subgroup. This becomes a priority simply due to the high prevalence of this directional preference subgroup coupled with their highly favorable outcomes using directional self-care determined by the assessment findings.

The decision of how best to provide this MDT evaluation for Sue is of great importance and is covered in Chapter 13. Any compromise in the expertise of this evaluation in turn compromises your understanding of Sue's low back problem. For example, should Sue have a directional preference and be a centralizing patient but remains undetected due to an inadequate MDT exam, she is not only deprived of the opportunity to recover quickly, simply, and inexpensively, her risk of undergoing unnecessary diagnostic and treatment interventions rises significantly. At least some of these consequences are expensive, some very expensive, and some even involve health risks.

Let's look at two common but opposite scenarios for Sue.

Scenario 1: If a reliable MDT exam determined that Sue does in fact have a directional preference, which means a direction of end-range movement that centralizes and even abolishes her pain, your clinical decisions are greatly simplified, but her management to lead her to full recovery of all her activities requires expert guidance.

Her initial treatment has already been objectively determined by these findings; the treatment also provides high expectations of a good-to-excellent recovery if Sue complies with her directional self-care instructions to control her pain. While no published data support this, widespread clinical experience indicates that full recoveries are much more likely if her care is guided by a well-trained MDT clinician. That might be you, if you have undergone such training, or a therapist or chiropractor to whom you have referred Sue.

Her ability to continue her work and recreational activities would quickly be determined by her ability to control, eliminate, and keep her symptoms from returning. If she gains control quickly, she might not need to miss any work at all, but will likely need to perform some simple exercises intermittently at work. This all requires teaching Sue how to assess and bring about her own success in first eliminating and then preventing her symptoms, hence taking control of her underlying pain-generator. By quickly learning how to do that, she can guide herself in providing her back disorder with the circumstances it needs to fully heal and recover. The MDT clinician and her pain responses both have very important roles in her education.

Like most with a directional preference, Sue would be expected to gain control of, and even eliminate, her pain fairly quickly. Consequently, there is no need for any medications, certainly no prescription meds, and never any narcotics. For family medicine physicians, this latter point is especially valuable as they contemplate the long-term management of these patients in their practice. There is likewise no need for additional testing such as x-rays, advanced imaging (CTs, MRIs, or discograms), or EMGs, even if she presented with sciatica and neurological deficit, for these symptoms and signs are already reversing since the directional means of reversing her pain and underlying problem have now been identified during her assessment.

It is also important for Sue to learn and understand that it is insufficient for her to merely abolish her pain. Abolishing the pain is actually only the first of three stages of her recovery. I routinely state: "the pain going away does not mean the problem has gone away."

Patients like Sue often complete this first stage fairly quickly, but must then quickly learn the importance of keeping her pain from returning by becoming proactive with her exercises, rather than just reactive to her pain. This protects her still recovering underlying disorder from those mechanical stresses that would begin to reverse it again, allowing her symptoms to recur. To remain pain-free, Sue must continue to provide her underlying disorder with both the time and opportunity to heal or stabilize itself, not unlike the need to protect a skin cut from further trauma or with a bandage so it can completely heal, even though the pain from that laceration has subsided.

It is imperative that you and Sue realize why her pain is now gone. It is not because she has fully recovered, for she can bring her pain back quite quickly. She is rather pain-free because of the directional changes she has been making in her life that her pain source appreciates. But her pain source is still there. She has simply learned to control it so it is not be causing further pain at the moment. Now in Stage 2 of her recovery, she must continue to perform her exercises, no longer because she is in pain, but because she doesn't want her pain to return. This then provides her pain source with the environment and conditions it needs to recover and heal.

I have always found analogies to be helpful to many patients, and there are plenty of them. If, for example, we knew little about how cars work, we might soon run out of gas because we didn't know to fill the tank. So we first learn to fill the tank *in reaction to* the car ceasing to run. But to avoid running out of gas again, we must now learn to put gas in proactively, not reactively. We must interrupt our busy schedule to stop, often somewhat inconveniently, at the gas station to put gas in our car, not because it's run out of gas, but because we don't want it to.

Likewise, people understand the need to continue to wear an un-wanted cast on their broken leg long after the pain has gone away because the broken bone needs time and opportunity for healing to take place. Taking the cast off before the bone is healed, perhaps justified just be-cause the pain is gone, allows the unhealed bone to come apart again and the pain returns. We must then re-apply the cast, again get rid of the pain and then move on to the important healing stage again.

Sue quickly learns that this is not just some theory for managing her pain. If she has not fully recovered yet, all she need do is try some excessive forward bending or prolonged slouched sitting, usually just inadvertently, and she will re-create the very pain she has been trying to eliminate from her life. Fortunately, she now knows what to do to reverse and eliminate her pain again, which provides her one more opportunity to use her newly learned exercise to eliminate her pain again that she also now realizes she has just brought back on herself. She now understands even better the rapid reversibility of her problem and the need for her to take better proactive control of her low back disorder so her recovery can progress.

In this Stage 2 of her recovery, Sue's underlying disorder must be provided the opportunity to heal and stabilize so her pain will no longer recur. In the case of treating the cut and the broken leg, healing can only happen if it is given the opportunity to do so. You recall Hippocrates line: "Healing is a matter of time, but it is also a matter of opportunity." This second stage of proactivity is Sue's healing or stabilizing stage. It may only take 1–2 days if the pain is of recent onset, but it might also take a week or more for those who begin this form of treatment after a much longer pain duration.

Of course, our ultimate goal is for Sue to return to all her prior activities; i.e., bending, lifting, sitting, work, and sports, without her pain returning. This is akin to the goal of returning the broken leg to walking, running and jumping. That "return-to-prior-activities process," often thought of as rehabilitation, is her third stage of care. But for Sue, it can't begin until sufficient healing has occurred in Stage 2 to withstand the added stress of forward bending. The cast can't come off the broken leg until sufficient healing has taken place, when the third stage can begin, the rehab stage if you will. It is here that one progressively puts more weight on the healing broken leg, at first still using crutches and then a cane, followed by full weight-bearing with limping, then walking, and finally running. The bone completes its full healing and strengthening as it is progressively challenged by those activities.

It is the same with Sue's back problem. It has been vulnerable to flexion from the outset. She has learned to successfully prevent her pain by avoiding flexion while using extension exercises, first reactively in Stage 1 and then proactively in Stage 2, to first centralize and abolish her pain, and then keep it from returning.

So the very question becomes: how soon can she begin to safely flex? After all, that is the goal of our treatment: returning her to all activities without pain. But how long must she avoid flexion and the risk of re-creating her pain? That answer is variable but fortunately the timing to begin flexion can quite safely be determined for each individual by slowly and progressively challenging the underlying disorder with flexion forces (a standard MDT protocol exists) while closely monitoring for any returning symptoms that would indicate that the underlying problem isn't ready yet.

In reality, this third stage often progresses quite quickly as long as symptoms do not recur, but it also sometimes can drag out, especially if Sue keeps trying to introduce too much flexion too soon. By monitoring for any return of symptoms during Sue's initial introduction of lumbar flexion and while progressively adding more and more flexion stress to the low back, Sue is able to track the readiness of her back disorder and safely progress back to all her flexion activities with no or few setbacks along the way.

Guided by experienced MDT clinicians, patients can often move themselves quite rapidly through these three stages to full recovery. However, if guided improperly to respect and self-manage these three stages, symptoms often keep recurring, even though the patient has learned well how to centralize and abolish them. I suspect that future research will demonstrate that understanding these management principles is one important reason why MDT-Credentialed clinicians are more successful in managing this directional preference subgroup than clinicians with less training. Treatment and recovery requires more than just performing an exercise that matches one's directional preference.

For those directional preference patients who have been symptomatic for months or years before finding out that they can centralize and abolish their pain, it may be useful beyond these three stages to address their overall physical deconditioning. Strengthening of lumbar musculature appears to be especially beneficial in these cases.

Such additional care is typically unnecessary in the recovery from acute and even subacute LBP. I would add that trying to treat acute LBP in someone with an undiscovered derangement by focusing on strengthening their trunk or lumbar musculature can be problematic. Indeed, 15% of those in the Long et al study treated with mid-range exercises reported their LBP worsened and dropped out of treatment.[90] Ignoring the mechanical needs of the acute pain source may be akin to attempting to use or strengthen muscles around a broken leg without first dealing with the underlying fracture itself.

Scenario 2: Alternatively, if Sue's MDT exam determines that she is *not* a member of the directional preference subgroup, there are pathways to consider that are also determined by other findings in her MDT exam.

First, during her MDT assessment, though she may not have a directional preference, she may still fall into the MDT derangement syndrome (see Chapter 7). This usually means she likely has a mechanically *irreversible* disc disorder of some sort; i.e., a painful protrusion, a sequestered fragment if she has sciatica as well, or a stubborn internal disc disorder (see Figure 9–2). Given the inability for the MDT assessment to identify a means of centralizing and abolishing her pain, all the usual diagnostic and therapeutic interventions associated with evaluating and managing a disc disorder come into play at this point. Todd Wetzel, MD, Professor of Orthopaedic and Neurosurgery at Temple University School of Medicine in Philadelphia, and I wrote an overview article on the management of disc patients using these MDT assessment methods at the outset of care that many have found useful in considering their clinical decision-making.[159] Identifying and eliminating from disc surgery consideration those found to have a directional preference, and those who can centralize and eliminate their own pain, should become everyone's top priority.

Another alternative is that Sue's low back problem may indeed be mechanical, but fit one of the other smaller MDT syndromes; i.e., Dysfunction or Postural (see Chapter 7 and Figure 9–2). Her treatment would then still be self-care and patient-specific, determined by the specific and reliable[76, 116] pattern of pain response elicited during her assessment. While there is evidence of reliability in identifying members of the postural and dysfunction syndromes, there have so far been no cohort predictive studies published focused on these two mechanical subgroups.

Finally, there are indeed patients who do have dominating psychosocial factors that truly are obstacles to their recovery and need to be addressed (see Figure 9–2). However, given the high prevalence of these easily and reliably identifiable MDT mechanical subgroups, along with the excellent prognosis of the very large directional preference subgroup, this psychosocially dominant subgroup is a great deal smaller than most clinicians and researchers would expect. It simply cannot, and should not, be positively identified until MDT is provided and completed.

More about strengthening the trunk musculature

Only one RCT has so far compared the benefits of the MDT method of care with that of an intensive dynamic strengthening program in treating chronic LBP.[111] In 260 consecutive patients, most of whom had experienced pain for longer than three months, MDT seemed equally effective as an intensive lumbar strengthening program in the treatment of patients with mostly chronic low back pain. With eight months of follow-up, this is a very respectable result for MDT given that the prevalence of directional preference and centralization would have fallen off considerably by the time patients' conditions become chronic.

What is not clear is whether these two interventions both recovered patients with similar mechanical conditions or each intervention provided benefit to dissimilar baseline mechanical conditions. If the latter, one chronic subgroup would have benefited and recovered using MDT and the other subgroup with strengthening and these two treatments would be used for distinctly different chronic LBP subgroups. This is another case of a black box study design that did not include such a subgroup analysis.

Chronic patients with a directional preference who can centralize and abolish their pain fairly quickly may not routinely need a purposeful formal rehabilitation program to help restore their ability to function fully. In a report published by the New Zealand Accident Compensation Corporation, chronically disabled LBP individuals who could significantly reduce, centralize or abolish their pain were able to return to normal activity and participate in their favorite sport without requiring any specific strengthening program.[33] Simply restoring their ability to move without pain enabled them to progressively return to their work and leisure activities, enabled them to restore any deconditioning and lost strength as their physical activity increased.

Unfortunately, there are no data as yet to help guide in which cases one can justify the added expense of a formal strengthening program. It is logical that some longer-term chronic LBP patients would benefit from a strengthening program, and there is good cohort data from such programs that do not commence with an MDT intervention that focus on isolating and strengthening the short extensors of the lumbar spine.[85, 108] These cohort studies used computerized dynamometers for isometric lumbar strengthening and not only report excellent strength gains, but also a decrease in recurrences and subsequent utilization of health care services.[85]

It should be noted that some of these training devices require the lumbar spine to "bend" to full or near end-range of both flexion and extension. The potential mechanical benefits of taking these motion segments, and in particular the discs, to end-range must also be taken into account as a possible contributor to pain reduction. Beyond these mechanical factors and the muscular strength gains themselves, other benefits may include improved lumbar circulation and neuromuscular facilitation as one initiates such a strengthening program.

"Core strengthening," often referred to as a "stabilization" program, is commonly advocated as the best primary treatment for most chronic LBP. It is also utilized by many MDT clinicians, but in a very selective and small subset of patients amongst those without a directional preference. However, there is little, if any, RCT evidence of its efficacy nor has there been adequate research into predicting who will and will not benefit from this form of care. It is clearly not necessary for everyone, but no studies to my knowledge have focused on the patient selection process. It is certainly unnecessary in most of the large group of acute and subacute LBP who are centralization/directional preference patients and do so well with directional end-range exercises and then return to normal activities. More long-term follow-up studies are needed of course, especially those that focus on recurrences and utilization of health care.

Given the growing data regarding the benefits of MDT for individuals with chronic LBP, it seems only logical that, if strengthening adds benefit in preventing recurrences, its place is as an adjunct or secondary intervention, always after the underlying mechanical characteristics are thoroughly evaluated and appropriately addressed. Alternatively, treating every chronic patient with strengthening, not an uncommon approach, without initially evaluating and treating the underlying mechanical problem, seems to me to be like proceeding directly to strengthening the thigh muscles associated with a fractured femur without first addressing the fracture, or ignoring the presence and care of an acutely torn knee meniscus by moving directly to strengthening the quads and hamstrings.

The Delitto classification system attempts to distinguish those acute patients who will receive benefit with core stabilization exercises from those with an extension directional preference who they feel should be treated with directional exercises. Their directional end-range testing however is significantly less thorough than the MDT assessment we've been describing so there are very likely undetected centralizers that land in their stabilization exercise program, thereby loosing the benefits of directly managing their overlooked reversible derangement.

For the much larger subgroup with a directional preference, there has been no research published that has addressed who might and might not benefit from strengthening of any type. Despite the fact that trunk and lumbar extensor strengthening is intuitively a beneficial thing, even for healthy individuals, there is insufficient data as to which patients, after eliminating their pain using the MDT approach, then either do or do not derive long-term benefit from a formal strengthening program. Clinical experience by MDT clinicians suggests that the progressive return to all pre-LBP activities while remaining pain-free is usually sufficient.

3. Predicting outcomes: obstacles and pathways to recovery:

the colored flag system

In Chapter 8, we discussed the numerous studies that document the excellent outcomes and recoveries of patients who have a directional preference and can centralize their pain. They can then treat themselves using directional exercises and matching postural strategies focused on controlling, eliminating, and then preventing their pain.

In contrast, as we just pointed out in the previous section, patients who are found to be non-centralizers, in whom no directional preference is identified during baseline assessment, usually have poor outcomes, regardless of their treatment. The absence of centralization during baseline assessment in an acute LBP subgroup was a far stronger predictor of either prolonged or non-recoveries than was the presence of any psychosocial factor.[157] Indeed, non-centralization was even a stronger predictor of poor outcomes than was centralization in predicting good outcomes.

Nevertheless, as discussed in Chapter 9, it's the psychosocial factors that have received so much attention in acute LBP clinical guidelines as potential "obstacles to recovery." Such factors are now commonly referred to as *yellow flags*, indicating the presence of psychosocial factors that might need attention if the patient is not recovering. Yellow flags, of course, perpetuate the colored flag theme that began with *red flags*, patient history elements that represent the possibility of some sinister etiology underlying the presenting back symptoms. These patients might have a spinal tumor, infection, inflammatory disease, some intra-abdominal cause, or cauda equina syndrome. All these red flags are in need of prompt specialized attention.

Over the past few years, at least two more colored flags have been described, each representing additional obstacles to recovery.[94] *Blue flags* are said to indicate the presence of negative perceptions or attitudes of workers with LBP toward their workplace environment while *black flags* represent systemic issues that affect the workplace, like the health care system itself and workers compensation features.

What is quite apparent from this expanding flag system is that the prevailing mindset, especially amongst primary care LBP researchers, is to focus on obstacles to recovery and return to productivity. But should we limit our focus accentuating the negative? As I pointed out in Chapter 9, there would no doubt be considerable value in studying and contemplating factors that instead lead to recovery. Why not at least contemplate the positive? For example, how do we explain recoveries that occur despite the presence of yellow, blue or black flags at baseline? A better understanding of the interaction between favorable and unfavorable predictors in the same patients would certainly provide some valuable insight to help us unlock some of the LBP mystery.

In that light, shouldn't we also be looking for *green flags*? A colleague of mine even suggested a checkered flag. But shouldn't we be looking for indicators or predictors of successful or excellent outcomes? Given the population data of a high persistence of symptoms one year after onset, we cannot count on a good prognosis based on the natural history of LBP.

Furthermore, given the high occurrence of excellent outcomes predicted for patients whose pain centralizes at baseline with a directional preference, these clinical findings represent a very legitimate and important green flag. This green flag is reliably identified and indicates the presence of a reversible underlying pain-generator. It may actually be the most important and valuable predictive flag of all. It is certainly the most prevalent, being elicited in 70% of acute and 50% of chronic LBP sufferers.

As I've already mentioned, when this green flag is found concurrently in someone who also has yellow flags, the predictive power of a poor result by the yellow flags disappeared from the findings of the regression analysis in the one study that directly analyzed the interaction between green and yellow flags.[157] To my knowledge, no data have been presented as yet pertaining to the interaction of this green flag (directional preference and centralization) with either blue or black flags, yet considerable anec-

> ## "Shouldn't we also be looking for *green flags*?"

dotal experience across MDT clinicians indicates that this green flag of reversibility is a strong predictor of return to work, even overcoming the negative influences of the workplace environment and occasionally even an adverse compensation system.

4. Understanding disease process

I began this book pointing out that our biggest dilemma is in not knowing where the pain is coming from in most LBP patients. The Quebec Task Force referred to this as the "fundamental source of error" . . . that "routinely introduces inaccuracies which are then further confounded with each succeeding step in care."

That dilemma has not, and will not, change in the near future if we continue to ignore LBP subgroup identification and validation using the A–D–T–O research model. If we learn only one thing from the past 30 years of black box RCTs, it is that continuance of such a focus will contribute little, if anything, to solving this problem.

More and more health care professionals, payers, employers, and patients are awakening to this reality. The times they are a-changin'. We have already made considerable progress in the minds of those who appreciate the substantial body of evidence that validates directional preference and centralization as characteristics of a large and important LBP subgroup. But, very importantly, in what way can these subgroups contribute to our quest to identify the source of pain in this very large subgroup?

To address that, let's be more specific with our question: why does centralization always occur with a single direction of end-range testing and then remain better when the test movements cease? The answer to this question will shed a great deal of light on the mechanism and source of pain production in this very large subgroup.

Fortunately, an anatomic diagnosis (or even theory) is unnecessary for successful MDT recoveries

Unlike most other LBP paradigms of care, MDT does not usually require one to determine or even speculate where the pain is coming from in order to select the best treatment. In contrast, most others systems base their treatment choices on unproven pain-generating theories and unreliable exam and imaging findings. In most cases, the selected treatment addresses their best theory of pain production rather than any objectively determined examination measures that characterize the nature of the patients' actual problems.

In contrast, MDT's simplicity is a large part of why it is so attractive. If you can affect the pain with end-range spinal loading tests, that is centralize, abolish, worsen or peripheralize it, you are very likely directly affecting its source, whatever that may be. Further, if a patient can abolish their pain using exercises that then enables them to get back to their activities (all part of the full MDT management of that patient), it really doesn't matter much where the pain was coming from. It's not necessary to know what it is to solve it, which is most fortunate since we have no way yet of finding out. But whatever it was, it's obviously been addressed. The only time it really matters where the pain is coming from is if some invasive treatment, like an injection or surgery, is being contemplated.

But where *is* that pain coming from?

In our quest to better understand why LBP occurs and why so many patients are centralizers with a directional preference, if nothing else, it is of immense academic interest to determine the underlying mechanism and anatomic source of pain in this very large subgroup.

We previously discussed the 1990 study as the first data presented on centralization where 98% of centralizers reported good or excellent outcomes at the conclusion of their care.[56] Another important point of interest in this study's data was that the small number of subjects who required disc surgery (N=4) were all non-centralizers when assessed at baseline. Upon imaging, three of those four had extruded discs while the fourth had no herniation but a positive discogram. All four had very good surgical outcomes. But note again that none of these surgical patients had a directional preference or could centralize their pain.

Like all good research, this raised another important research question: can this MDT form of assessment distinguish those with surgical disc pathology from those who can recover without surgery? Can it distinguish those with reversible, that is, reducible disc pathology from those whose disc pathology is irreversible or irreducible and therefore more likely to need surgery?

We'll return to this and other surgery-related questions shortly.

We know from Nachemson's early intradiscal pressure measurements that lumbar disc pressures increase when they are loaded in flexion such as with forward bending or slouched sitting and are then lowered when the spine is erect.[105] These elevated disc pressures with flexion have long been felt to explain why disc symptoms so commonly increase during flexion activities and positions. Unfortunately, the interest in full lumbar extension in those days was insufficient to prompt measurement of those pressures, either standing or prone.

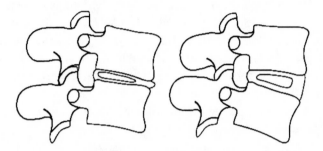

Figure 10–1: The intervertebral disc nucleus is under increased pressure and is moved toward the back of the disc (to the left in the left-hand figure) with forward bending and is under pressure and moves toward the front (to the right in the right-hand drawing) when we are erect and bend backward.

Subsequent biomechanical data support that peripheral disc loading associated with lumbar flexion and extension creates pressure gradients across the disc that move nuclear content away from that load (Figure 10–1).[58, 122, 125, 126, 128] This nuclear movement is a necessary response to spinal bending that enables discs to assume the required wedge-shape that allows the spine to flex, extend or side bend. The nuclei must move down the pressure gradient and out of the way for the adjacent vertebral margins to approximate on the concave side of the bend.

These disc mechanical characteristics beg the questions of whether or not this is the articular surface or mechanism that is directional and can become disrupted in McKenzie's derangement syndrome? Is this the reversible mechanism that malfunctions to cause the rapid changes in symptoms and range of motion that we elicit in directional preference patients? The evidence points that way.

If the annulus remains competent to maintain the disc's hydrostatic mechanism, the first relevant question becomes: can asymmetric disc loading from one direction of spinal bending be sufficient to cause pain-generating displacement of nuclear content on the opposite side of the disc? Based on known disc pain caused by nuclear protrusion, herniation and extrusion, the answer seems clear: Yes. But the second more provocative question then becomes: can this pain-generating displaced nuclear content be made to retreat or be reduced to its former, more central "home" by bending the spine to end-range in the opposite direction, creating an oppositely directed pressure gradient that enables decompression and relief of the stress that had been applied to the innervated annulus and/or nerve root by displaced nuclear content? Is the pain response of centralization a reflection of the relief of the pain-generating tissues from the offending displaced nuclear content being restored to its more normal location?

Michael Adams, Ph.D., Professor of Anatomy at the University of Bristol in England and one of the world's foremost disc and spinal biomechanical investigators, has extensively studied these pressure gradients and nuclear displacements.[2, 3] He has stated that LBP, with or without radiating leg pain, is commonly generated from excessive nuclear displacement sufficient to either mechanically or chemically irritate the innervated outer layers of the annulus, gaining access to those layers through a fissure or alternatively by causing an annular herniation that directly compresses an adjacent nerve root. He is quite familiar with the pain response of centralization and the MDT clinical methods and has stated at spine conferences and in a recent personal communication that he knew of no other explanation that better fits the phenomenon of pain centralization.

Evidence of unnecessary disc surgery!

Large numbers of LBP patients who are centralizers remain undetected. This is because either they are never provided the opportunity to undergo an MDT assessment or, if they were, the assessment was carried out in an inadequate or incomplete fashion due to incomplete examiner training. Consequently, their pain and disability often persists and, if at sufficient levels, they may end up undergoing unnecessary disc surgery. This is tragic. It is also obviously avoidable, even on a wide scale, if proper and thorough MDT evaluations were a routine, even required, part of "exhausting conservative care" prior to entertaining injections or surgery.

For economic reasons of course, no surgeon or his or her hospital wish to see their surgical volumes diminish, yet all agree that unnecessary surgery is to be avoided. So how often is this type of unnecessary surgery taking place?

First, let's recall the Long et al study in which patients were only randomized if they demonstrated a directional preference.[90] One-third of those patients had pain radiating below the knee and half of those had a mild neurological deficit, indicating these patients' pain was likely of disc origin. This entire directional preference group reported excellent recoveries in just two weeks when treated with matching directional exercises. Thus the critical question when evaluating each individual patient with sciatica becomes: does this disc pathology have a directional preference that can be utilized to bring about a rapid non-surgical recovery for this patient? In other words, is this a rapidly reversible, reducible derangement?

The importance of asking that question is illustrated in four prospective studies of patients who have reached the point in their care where disc surgery was being contemplated.[50, 80, 82, 115] With an insufficient response to non-operative care, patients typically then undergo MRIs and often invasive discography to evaluate a suspected lumber disc herniation or an internal disc disorder. If a disc source for their pain is identified, a surgical procedure is often recommended and carried out, at substantial expense with the usual risk of complications with the possibility of only producing temporary or limited or no improvement, and even worsening of the situation (failed back syndrome). Some speculate that the surgeon's understanding of the potential downsides of surgical treatment explains why, when asked what treatments they would choose for their own LBP, they are typically reluctant to choose surgery. So the stakes are very high for patients and payers alike at this critical decision point in LBP management.

The first study focused on patients with sciatica and neurological loss who were being considered for disc surgery.[80] Although published way back in 1986, it has unfortunately been under most everyone's radar largely because it is "only" a cohort study. But it has a most important and provocative message for all LBP stakeholders. It reported on 67 patients with sciatica, positive neurological findings, and blocked lumbar extension motion, who were experiencing no improvement with extensive outpatient care. Admitted to the hospital for consideration of disc surgery, they were fortunate that their doctors had heard about the McKenzie extension exercises that were thought to maybe restore displaced disc content to its normal position. Each patient was therefore instructed to perform prone passive lumbar extension tests (Figure 7–2) within the limits of their available range and pain tolerance to see what would happen. Just over half (52%) reported that their pain did not worsen as a result of this testing and were therefore instructed to perform sets of extension exercises (Figure 7–2) several times a day over the next few days of their hospitalization.

Within 2–5 days, every one of these patients experienced a rapid reversal of their painful condition. They all regained their full extension range of motion while completely resolving their symptoms, thereby eliminating any need for surgery. In contrast, all but one of the other 48% whose pain was aggravated with the initial extension testing underwent surgical removal of their herniated disc. Most were found to have either free disc fragments in their spinal canal or swollen nerve roots from their herniations.

If these patients had not been given the opportunity to undergo this testing, most, if not all, would likely have undergone unnecessary surgery. That was 52% of their surgical candidates.

There are two additional points about this study worth considering. First, how many more could have also avoided surgery if their doctors had known to test them in other directions besides just extension. Data from other studies suggest there may have been 5–10 more who would have a *lateral* directional preference and who also could have recovered without surgery. Secondly, a subsequent paper reported that, of the patients located five years later who had recovered so quickly without surgery, none had required subsequent surgery.[5]

The other two pertinent studies reported on patients without surgical discs evident on their MRIs but who then underwent discography to evaluate the presence or absence of internal disc pathology at the point in their care when they were being considered for some type of intra-discal procedure, fusion, or disc arthroplasty.[50, 82] Both study protocols required them to undergo an MDT exam immediately prior to their discogram.

Despite this relatively late point in their care, the percentages of patients whose pain responded with a centralization pattern in these two studies were 49% and 32% respectively. While no follow-up was reported in either study (both papers focused only on the correlation between the results of the MDT and discography assessments), there is ample evidence in seven cohort and four RCT studies that most in this centralization subgroup do very well with non-surgical treatment consisting of directional exercises and posture strategies.

Once again, a substantial percentage of pre-surgery patients were found to be previously undetected centralizers.

The fourth study reported the effect on disc surgery rates of introducing Mechanical Diagnosis and Therapy (McKenzie care) in patients with sciatica for greater than one month.[115] Starting in 1997, the general practitioners in one county in Denmark began referring these patients to one of two new spine clinics where MDT played a prominent role. That county's first time disc surgery rates decreased by two-thirds over the next four years while surgical rates across the rest of Denmark were unchanged over that same time period.

These four studies should be of immense interest to all LBP patients and clinicians contemplating disc surgery, as well as employers or payers who pay for these procedures. It is also noteworthy that, due to the almost exclusive focus on black box RCTs by guideline panels or other literature reviewers, these very important cohort studies have been completely overlooked.

The first three of these studies were reviewed in some detail, along with disc physiology and mechanical studies, in the peer-reviewed journal article I mentioned earlier by Dr. Todd Wetzel and me. This article also described the use of the MDT form of assessment as the basis for managing symptomatic lumbar disc disease.[159] The paper's most compelling point, and the obvious take-away message from all these studies, is that *the evidence is sufficiently strong that LBP patients should not be undergoing disc surgery of any type without first being given the opportunity to be evaluated using this simple and inexpensive form of assessment.* The routine pre-operative selection process, which always follows the mantra of "exhausting all conservative care," should routinely include this assessment and will at some point, I have no doubt, be required by payers as part of their authorization process.

The most expensive and unfortunate centralizers are those that are never discovered. And that happens every day in every city and town, and in every clinic where LBP patients are not provided this evaluation by a clinician sufficiently trained in these techniques.

5. LBP primary and secondary prevention

> *When you hear something, you forget it;*
> *when you see something, you remember it;*
> *when you do something, you understand it.*
> —*Chinese Proverb*

Primary LBP prevention

The primary prevention of LBP means preventing it from ever happening in the first place. Most believe this form of prevention is a long way off, if it is even possible. LBP is such a ubiquitous part of life, yet perhaps certain lifestyle and furniture design alterations will some day prove to be effective. But, realistically, who would be sufficiently motivated to alter their lifestyle in any way in order to prevent the pain of something they had never before experienced? Very few I think. Yet, the data say that 20% never experience LBP throughout life. Why is that subgroup able to avoid such pain? Maybe it's genetic. Yet, to date, there is no evidence that LBP can be intentionally primarily prevented.

Secondary LBP prevention

Secondary prevention is another matter however. This refers to preventing recurrences after the initial episode. In light of how commonly LBP recurs, and especially if recurrences progressively worsen, as we discussed in Chapter 4, this is of course a very relevant topic.

One RCT evaluated the use of MDT principles in an effort to achieve both primary and secondary prevention success.[81] A sizeable number of healthy military recruits in Denmark are normally expected to experience and seek care for LBP during their ten months of strenuous basic training. A sample of these recruits were randomly assigned to either no intervention or some initial training and instruction in performing one session of press-ups every day (Figure 7–2) with daily exercise compliance mandated by their commanding officer. They were also taught to focus on sitting erectly rather than slouched.

For the group using extension exercises and sitting more erectly, LBP reporting was reduced significantly (only 33% of recruits versus 51% in the control group, p<.009) as was consulting the regiment infirmary for low back care (9% versus 25%, p<.002). However, in those who had never experienced back pain before, there was only a small difference in outcomes. So secondary prevention was much more successful than primary prevention. Perhaps there was better compliance with the intervention from those who had prior experience with LBP.

Knowing the large size of the subset of LBP with a directional preference for extension, it should not be surprising that a prevention program emphasizing more extension and less flexion might be helpful. Further studies may yet show some primary prevention benefit using an extension-oriented approach that addresses and counteracts the human species's flexed lifestyle of sitting and forward bending.

Of course, with such a favorable view of the natural history of LBP and little apparent awareness that recurrent episodes ever worsen, until recently, there's been little attention directed toward secondary prevention on the part of guideline panels. The only effort has been the European

Guidelines for Prevention of Low Back Pain published in 2004.[21] Not surprisingly, their primary preventive recommendation was to perform physical exercise, with no specific type recommended.

Interestingly, the Danish military recruit study, though cited in this guideline, "did not alter the conclusions" of the guideline, implying that the extension exercise intervention in that study was simply lumped into the guidelines' general recommendation of physical exercise. There was again a clear lack of understanding of the preventive benefit that these simple extension exercises added over and above the benefits of general physical exercise, which was the alternate treatment intervention in the study. After all, how much more vigorous can exercise be than to engage in nine months of basic military training? Could this study have been reviewed by those with an established notion (bias?) that only general exercise was of value with no additional benefit from any specific form of exercise?

But let's get back to natural history where we have already discussed population data that: 1) many LBP sufferers remain symptomatic with activity restrictions one year later, and 2) for many who experience recurrences, their episodes become progressively more severe.[54, 152, 153]

One additional provocative pilot study[140] reported data regarding secondary prevention and showed that a chronic LBP cohort that averaged more than four episodes of LBP in the year prior to the study, after reading McKenzie's patient-focused book *Treat Your Own Back*,[102] significantly reduced their recurrences over the following 18 months. Specifically, between 9 and 18 months after reading the book, subjects reported a 95% reduction in recurrent episodes which subjects attributed to the exercises they were performing and posture modifications made as a result of reading the book. While this study had no control group, such a dramatic reduction in pain and recurrences is not inconsistent with the results of other studies, including the Long et al RCT.[90] But it has, not surprisingly, been overlooked in preventive LBP discussions and reviews because it has no control group. Again, more research is needed but such results should encourage researchers to focus on the potential to prevent recurrences using MDT methods of self-care.

Let me add that my own 20-year experience using MDT methods, which also parallels the experience of every MDT-trained clinician I know, allows me to make what I feel is a safe prediction. Once clinical studies begin to routinely monitor recurrences as one of their outcome measures, objective data will emerge that document what directional preference patients have told us over and over again: "That exercise you taught me last year that eliminated my pain continues to be very useful." They then add one of two things. They either say: 1) as long as I perform my exercises regularly, I have had no further back pain episodes (pro-active exercise use); or 2) whenever my pain returns, I can always eliminate it by performing that exercise (reactive exercise use). But whether they are exercising proactively or reactively, this large subgroup are very grateful for their ability to prevent their prior episodes that plagued them with all sorts of difficulties for so long.

Indeed, MDT clinicians are so aware of the value of teaching patients how to prevent recurrences, one of their top priorities during their initial patient assessment, as they identify directional mechanical factors that bring on patients' current pain, is to correlate them with the circumstances patients recall that led to prior episodes. These are invariably consistent with one another and begin to point to the directional self-care strategies that will assist in preventing future episodes. Based on their patients' feedback, most of these clinicians are convinced that successfully addressing recurrence prevention ultimately provides the best long-term outcome for each individual patient.

6. Cost reduction: the problem of the high cost of low back care

Throughout health care in the U.S., both the historical focus and the economic profit have been in treating disease, not in maintaining health. Many feel that these two are inexorably linked, always being in a reactive mode to disease and health crises, rather than being proactive or preventative. Health care systems historicallyl struggled with spending a few dollars upfront to save large amounts later by avoiding or minimizing disease and its complications.

One bright light is the notion of disease management, a growing health care industry that is making a major effort to provide proactive programs by encouraging better patient self-care and treatment compliance. I'll discuss this further later in this chapter.

Our predominant health care and reimbursement approach in medicine in general and for LBP in particular, is to minimize acute treatment, withholding resources until the consequences require high-priced specialists. Current LBP guidelines clearly portray this theme: minimize care for acute LBP by encouraging patients to remain active, with the intent of addressing the consequences for those whose pain becomes chronic. We are banking so heavily on LBP's natural history (see Chapter 4), viewed by most influential experts as being so favorable in bringing about widespread recovery, yet we are then spending exorbitant amounts on evaluating and treating the complications of non-recovery. We must learn more about the link between acute and chronic pain. But I digress.

In the U.S., health care costs are a huge part of the current threat to the very survival of large employers. These large employers bear the brunt of this high cost of low back care. Based on actual employer data I've reviewed, large self-insured U.S. companies with 100,000 or more employees may spend $30–40 million per year just for LBP. That's nearly $3,000 per individual with LBP or $300–400 per year for every single employee, even if they never have LBP. Other estimates are as high as $8,000 per LBP case.[107] The aggregate cost of low back care in the U.S. is often estimated at over $50 billion per year, with one 1998 analysis reporting it to be over $90 billion.[92]

As discussed in Chapter 2, commonly used LBP clinical assessments and patient classifying efforts are often driven by clinicians' unproven pain-generating theories, so clinical decision-making becomes very subjective and patient management highly variable and expensive. These high costs arise from excessive use of unnecessary, very often expensive, and, too often, ineffective treatments. Additionally, we must acknowledge the effect of patients concluding that they must have something seriously wrong, not always the case, based on the actions of their trusted practitioners who prescribe so many tests, treatments, and procedures.

It is important to realize that LBP clinicians get paid far more handsomely to investigate and treat the complications of LBP using hi-tech imaging, surgery, spinal implants, artificial discs, injections, and multi-disciplinary rehab programs, than to take proactive steps to avoid crises and complications. We will discuss shortly how payers might get far greater return for their money by being more proactive with LBP by implementing evidence-based care, in this case distinct from guideline-based care, when patients seek help acutely.

We should also acknowledge the potential savings by simply complying with current one-size-fits-all guideline recommendations. Catching the "low hanging fruit" of those who will recover regardless of their care without spending money on them unnecessarily can save money. This begs the question of whether that is really our most cost-effective care? And perhaps more importantly, is such an approach even realistic, given the pain and distress experienced by most individuals who seek care from clinicians who then respond by providing their best care for their needy patients? That "best care" again typically flows from the theories of the LBP generation in which each clinician was educated. This brings us back to the Tension Cycle introduced and discussed in Chapter 3.

Three cost-saving scenarios

Although no formal cost-effectiveness studies have been completed for MDT as yet, they will no doubt be forthcoming. In the meantime, the consistently positive outcome data generated from so many prospective cohort studies,[56, 65, 72, 88, 90, 129, 136, 157, 158] further re-enforced by the findings of four RCTs,[17, 18, 90, 121] carry strong implications for the potential positive effect on both direct and indirect costs of low back care if MDT is implemented.

If you wish, return to Chapter 8 to review these studies. They are also summarized in the Appendix. Recall that the Long et al study reported that 74% of those presenting with acute, subacute and chronic back pain were found during their baseline assessment to have a green flag; that is, a directional preference. When this large subgroup was randomized, 95% of those who performed exercises that directionally matched their directional preference improved or fully recovered in just two weeks, with no one worsening or withdrawing. These statistically significant and strongly positive outcomes were in remarkable contrast with the outcomes of subjects randomized to guideline-consistent care consisting of assurance of recovery, advice to remain active, and non-specific exercises, where only 42% improved or recovered. Fifteen percent actually worsened and 33% withdrew during treatment due to little or no improvement.

To understand the economic effect of all this, let's consider three clinical scenarios where MDT might be implemented. In the first, MDT assessment is implemented at the heart of our current crisis management model, at a critical decision-making point where costs and outcomes hang heavily in the balance. We'll then transition to two other strategic opportunities to use MDT in a more proactive way.

1. Eleventh hour pre-surgical rescues

Let's return our attention to that relatively small, yet very important and potentially expensive subset of LBP patients who have arrived at a critical, high stakes decision point in their care that is challenging to the patient, the provider, and the payer. I call this the eleventh hour scenario, when either disc excision or fusion surgery are being contemplated and often recommended.

We just reviewed three relevant studies that focused on this precise crisis point in care.[50, 80, 82] In all three, an MDT evaluation was provided to these patients at the eleventh hour (at (1) in Figure 10-2), just before surgery, with a sizable number (32–52%) reporting the green flag of centralization and directional preference when evaluated using the MDT assessment.

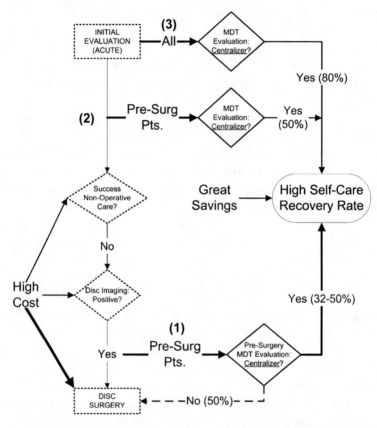

Figure 10–2: The conventional clinical sequence for LBP non-recoveries (shown in the left-hand column of dotted figures) often leads to disc surgery. Inserting a pre-surgical MDT evaluation at (1) instead finds as many as 50% of surgical candidates are undetected centralizers, most likely able to recover without surgery, with huge cost savings.

Even greater savings are available if those same patients were to instead undergo their MDT evaluation at the outset of their care, at (2), when their same recoveries would enable the avoidance of the cost of all their failed non-operative care, all their pre-surgical diagnostics, and again surgery.

For maximum savings, if all LBP patients underwent an MDT evaluation at the outset of their care, then in addition to the pre-surgical group, as many as 80% of all acute patients would be centralizers who, if managed properly, would be expected to avoid all subsequent costs of unnecessary non-operative care, diagnostic studies, surgery, chronic pain and disability.

Please understand that, in all three of these studies, surgery would have otherwise been performed in most patients. Most patients naturally would prefer to avoid surgery if they could instead experience a rapid recovery using some simple exercises and work on their posture. While surgeons and their hospitals would both be concerned about the lost income from fewer surgical procedures, it is their even stronger priority to avoid performing unnecessary surgery.

> "All of these undetected centralizers were also undetected centralizers during their first hour of care."

Of course, payers also substantially benefit by identifying centralizers at this eleventh hour, thereby eliminating $15,000–$40,000 for each avoided surgery, not including the additional costs related to incomplete recoveries, continued disabilities, complications, and second, even third, surgeries. How satisfying it is for all, particularly at this eleventh hour, to bring such simple resolution of both the physical and economic pain experienced by the patient and payer respectively?

Intervening with an MDT assessment at this critical time is a straightforward intervention requiring only a minor shift in thinking. Fortunately, for most, this is an easy shift consistent with all parties interest in "exhausting all conservative care" as a pre-requisite for performing any disc surgery.

Of course, without this means of subgrouping patients into centralizers and non-centralizers, payers find themselves stuck, at the mercy of the one-size-fits-all guideline recommendations and forced to spend large sums of money on avoidable non-operative and surgical procedures for undetected centralizers.

2. These undetected pre-surgical centralizers were centralizers from symptom onset

Let's now re-consider this same eleventh hour scenario by turning the clock back. All of these undetected centralizers were also undetected centralizers during their first hour of care (see (2) in Figure 10–2). Their pain would have centralized and abolished just as easily, often more easily, at the outset of their care when they could have also been guided to rapid recoveries using the directional preference treatment principles we've discussed.

Such an early recovery means that, in addition to their opportunity to again avoid their disc surgery, both payers and patients could have been spared all their pre-surgical interventions and costs, including all the medications, extensive physical therapy, chiropractic, or alternative and behavioral medicine care, as well as other specialist referrals. Their expensive MRIs and CTs would have also been unnecessary as well as any epidural and other forms of injections. The benefits also include the avoidance of the weeks or months of disruption in their quality of life and any lost work time and productivity.

Although these cost savings are only seen in retrospect, this same line of thinking reinforces the value of implementing MDT assessment at the outset of low back care to search for a green flag and to appreciate the immense cost-savings from avoiding all or most of these interventions that too often lead to the need for surgical decision-making.

3. The benefits of early MDT assessment[24]

Let's continue this same line of thought as we explore how to provide maximum savings for patient and payer alike by introducing MDT assessment routinely for all patients when first seeking care for their LBP (see (3) in Figure 10-2). Not surprisingly, advocating a single form of assessment for all LBP patients is unconventional, but the evidence and potential savings speak for themselves.

First, consider that introducing MDT early, focusing specifically on assessment and diagnosis, is in compliance with guideline recommendations that focus on self-care. As pointed out earlier, nothing is more reassuring of recovery for both patient and clinician than to learn very early how they can actually abolish and eliminate their own pain using some simple, yet specific, exercises. Furthermore, nothing is better at enabling patients to return to, or maintain, their work and activities than to help them rapidly reverse their problem by centralizing and abolishing their own pain, rather than aggravating it, and then also learn how to prevent its return. After all, if guidelines recommend searching for yellow flags in acute LBP patients, shouldn't they also recommend a search for green flags, since the presence or absence of green flags appears to be at least as strong, or even stronger, predictor of outcomes than the presence of yellow flags?[156]

Let's consider the benefits of implementing the MDT assessment early in one's low back care. Recall that, although the prevalence of centralization and directional preference may only be 32–52% in chronic and pre-surgical patients,[50, 80, 82, 88, 90] these green flags are elicited in 70–85% of individuals with acute LBP.[37, 56, 72, 90, 129, 136, 158] That discrepancy in percentages suggests that the pain generator in some patients actually loses its reversibility over time. Recall the deterioration of the pain source over the course of many recurrences was discussed in Chapter 4 as an important pathway between acute and chronic LBP as part of the natural history of LBP. In other words, if the problem is not prevented so recurrences continue, the episodes become progressively longer and worse until finally recovery no longer occurs because the pain generator has lost its ability to reverse, either rapidly or slowly, even in the hands of well-trained MDT practitioners.

A common clinical indication of such deterioration is contained in the patient histories of those whose pain is both chronic, often constant, and irreversible. Chronic patients with no current detectable directional preference commonly report that weeks or months earlier their pain was in fact intermittent, not yet constant. They also reported that, for a considerable period of time during this episode, their pain always worsened with lumbar flexion activities and positions and felt much better, even abolishing, with upright standing, walking or erect sitting.

In other words, historically, their early pain pattern revealed the directional preference green flag where intermittent pain was the rule, increasing with one direction of testing (usually flexion) and then centralizing or turning off with the opposite direction of testing (usually upright or extension). Patients with such a clear directional preference *history* invariably demonstrate that very same directional preference when they then perform repeated end-range *test movements*. For this chronic group however, in whom the pain no longer responds in this fashion, the pain generator responsible for the earlier reversible directional preference pain pattern has apparently now deteriorated to where it is now constant, the green flags of centralization and directional preference can no longer be elicited, and reduction of their derangement is no longer possible.

In reality however, as we know from the abundant prevalence data on centralization, when properly examined, 70% of acute LBP patients are centralizers with a directional preference but most of these in the general population are never discovered because they are never provided the opportunity to be appropriately assessed. Fortunately, whereas this assessment does require clinical expertise in order to minimize the likelihood of missing centralizers, this is not an expensive, high-tech assessment. Consider that a sizeable number of undetected acute centralizers, instead of rapidly recovering with appropriate MDT treatment, are at risk for non-recovery and creating all the quality of life and expense issues we have been discussing.

Despite the fact that the data show that treatment based on a patient's directional preference leads to excellent recoveries, it is also clear now that centralizers do not necessarily have good recoveries if they are not treated in this way. What seems readily apparent is that there are far greater savings for both patients and payers if the MDT assessment and care are made available at the outset of LBP care-seeking rather than waiting until patients are either chronic or pre-operative.

> Just because patients have reversible disorders does not mean they will reverse on their own, without MDT treatment. There's now plenty of data on chronic LBP patients found to be centralizers who obviously had not recovered previously with non-directional treatments.[50, 80, 82, 88, 90] This illustrates the great value of implementing MDT early.

Thus, MDT's most positive effect in terms of cost reduction can be distilled with a single key strategy:

As early as possible, all LBP patients should be provided the opportunity to be assessed by well-trained MDT clinicians to enable reliable classification into a validated subgroup.

Assessment-guided, patient-specific self-care usually then produces rapid recoveries because of the rapidly reversible nature of most LBP sources.

7. Disease management and low back care innovations

I believe the disease management industry deserves special mention here. Again, disease management focuses on developing and implementing programs to enable individuals with chronic diseases to better self-manage and comply with prescribed care in an effort to save the high costs of complications from their diseases. Prevalent diseases such as diabetes, hypertension, various forms of heart disease, asthma, renal failure are but a few of the many types served by disease management programs.

Because LBP so nicely fits this disease management profile of target diseases, there are immense opportunities to help employers and other payers avoid the high costs of non-recovery. A disease management program based on the MDT model is a natural fit enabling the majority of LBP individuals to access subgroup-specific self-care. Disease management companies now have the opportunity to offer *individualized*, evidence-based, self-care programs rather than a meager guideline-based program that only offers one-size-fits-all care.

Please permit a short commercial message here. I have led a team that has created a web-based patient educational program that is based on MDT principles. It:

1. first determines who can and can't benefit from pursuing this approach, then
2. teaches qualified individuals how to self-assess their own LBP, and then, because of its strong interactivity
3. uses participants' reported assessment findings to select the appropriate instructional content for teaching how to best centralize, abolish and finally prevent their own LBP.

This program, called "BackFix®" interfaces with disease management's widely used telephonic model to enhance the quality of the educational content while reducing the need for expensive telephone time to determine and then deliver individualized patient education. Leveraging both web technology and the quality of MDT content will enable disease management companies to assume an increased portion of risk in their interactions with their large self-insured employer clients.

Chapter 11

Goldmine Research Strategies and Projects

The goldmine implications for LBP research into subgroups are sufficient to warrant a chapter of their own. As evidence supporting the validation of these pain response subgroups grows and becomes more widely appreciated, each of the major areas of LBP management and understanding I've presented all represent research goldmines in need of exploration to uncover what many predict will significantly affect our approach to managing this $90 billion health care challenge.

Although there are many research questions to be asked, in essence subgroup-focused research will generally address two broad questions: In what ways are members of any particular subgroup unique from non-members? And are there then subgroup-specific treatments that enhance outcomes?

We need to study recoveries, not just failures to recover

In addition to systematic reviews and guidelines being fixed on black box RCTs, another unfortunate focus has been on identifying obstacles to recovery and why patients become chronic. While there is value in exploring these obstacles, an even more revealing area of investigation has been essentially ignored. As I stated earlier, we will not solve the mystery of LBP until we begin to analyze what goes right with recoveries. One of the most important, yet ignored, keys to understanding LBP is analyzing recoveries themselves.

Let me illustrate. Why do so many LBP sufferers recover, at least in the short run, on their own with what we refer to as "natural history," as discussed in Chapter 9? And why is the large directional preference subgroup such a bright green flag?

Of course we know from multiple studies that these two are not necessarily linked, otherwise those chronic patients found so late to be centralizers would have recovered by natural history long ago.[80, 88, 90] Even though they were centralizers, they had not recovered on their own or with any other treatment. Yet once correctly identified using the MDT assessment, proper MDT treatment obviously led to excellent outcomes. We must also consider that some of these patients' low back disorders were actually aggravated by their other treatments, as documented in the 2004 Long et al study where 15% of directional preference patients treated with evidence-based care actually worsened.[90]

So do these various forms of recovery have anything in common to help us better understand the onset and resolution of LBP episodes? And what about the dynamics of recurrences? If more than 50% of those with recurrences find their episodes progressively worsen over time, it is a significant contribution to learn how to resolve the current episode that then further provides insight into why the pain keeps recurring, and how to prevent this from happening.[54, 55]

Implementing the A–D–T–O model

We've learned so little from the past 25 years of black box RCTs that the Quebec Task Force's 1987 statements still apply: "There is so much variability in making a diagnosis that this initial step routinely introduces inaccuracies which are then further confounded with each succeeding step in care." The resulting diagnosis "is the fundamental source of error."

Spratt obviously agrees, but he has added a very constructive next step by describing how subgroup identification and validation research can and should be carried out.[133] He, in my opinion, correctly points out that, unless we adopt an A–D–T–O research strategy, we will be left with "articles written in another 25 years that suggest that Nachemson's (1976) lament that 85% of patients with low back pain have no specific diagnosis remains as true then as it was 50 years before."

Although it is true that many international experts advocate the importance of identifying subgroups and performing subgroup-focused RCTs,[14, 15, 36, 133] the folly of conducting black box RCTs over the years escapes them, as does the need to abandon this form of RCT. To get off this unproductive playing field, we must first establish the A–D and D–T links that then enable the performance of subgroup- or classification-based RCTs.

One of the inherent strengths of the A–D–T–O model is its more formal recognition of the value of non-RCT studies, in great contrast to most LBP clinical guidelines. RCTs are simply the wrong study design to establish either the A–D or D–T links yet they remain essential in validating LBP subgroups.

As part of the widespread implementation of the A–D–T–O research model, proponents of all LBP treatments, whether manual, exercise, modalities, injections, surgery, or whatever, will at some point be compelled to re-evaluate their existing research in the context of this model and then initiate the appropriate study designs in the hopes of eliminating current deficiencies. For the great majority of treatments, that deficiency starts with reliability studies in identifying the subgroup that will and won't respond well to each treatment.

New areas of research

There is so much productive research that will emerge as awareness of, and interest in, this form of MDT assessment grows. The centralization and directional preference subgroup, as a green flag, is particularly fascinating and informative in light of its high prevalence and strong prognostic character. I'd like to offer some research questions to ponder that should contribute to the "goldmine" of research tied to uncovering subgroups, disease process, clinical decision-making, and therefore cost savings.

1. Collaborative research between MDT and non-MDT clinical groups who have their own means of patient assessment and subgroup classification will be very informative and meaningful. To do so however, each system must first provide its own evidence for reliability in identifying subgroups.

One emerging LBP classification system has been developed by Anthony Delitto, PT, Ph.D., Chairman of the Physical Therapy Department at the University of Pittsburgh.[38, 65] This system emphasizes the importance of identifying distinct LBP subgroups that respond best to subgroup-specific treatments and is referred to as a "treatment-based" classification. It focuses on common treatments for LBP to see what baseline characteristics typify patients who experience good results from the various treatments in the system. As the system has evolved, the subgroups have diminished in number to where there are currently only three treatment-based subgroups of patients. These investigators have sought to identify "clinical prediction rules" whereby the identification of individual patient baseline characteristics make it more likely that they will respond to particular interventions.

An important feature of this system is its recognition of the evidence supporting the use of directional exercises found at baseline to centralize and abolish radiating LBP. However, these clinicians have not availed themselves of any formal MDT education. Early descriptions had patients perform only a single flexion and a single extension movement in search of centralization. Their examination protocol has evolved to where it incorporates repeated end-range movements, but it still limits their assessment to only flexion and extension test movements, overlooking all those who require lateral or rotational tests to elicit centralization. It is also likely that even their evaluation of flexion and extension testing is not nearly as thorough as it could be.

In that light, a common early deficiency during most clinicians' MDT learning curve is the lack of appreciation for the need to have patients move to their full end-range in any one direction, and performing it repetitively, before drawing conclusions about the effect of that direction of testing. Many centralizers are missed by repetitive directional tests that don't fully explore the available end-range. This also means that some centralizers may well be misclassified into other Delitto categories. This may explain why their published data report a far lower prevalence for centralization than what has been reported in the long list of studies in which MDT-trained clinicians conducted the assessments. No doubt the true prevalence of centralization is also influenced by its operational definition, which may also differ between the MDT and Delitto clinicians.

What is the right prevalence for centralization? Some collaborative research would be very helpful. Over-reporting of centralization by Credentialed MDT clinicians seems far less likely than under-reporting by the Delitto group, given the consistency of the high prevalence reported in so many MDT clinical studies with high Kappa values for inter-examiner reliability (k = .51 to 1.0).[4] Delitto clinicians' reliability for detecting centralization has been reported to be much lower (Kappa values = .15 to .55)[62] just as their centralization prevalence has been low.

2. Excellent collaborative research of another type has already taken place and there's so much more to do. Two studies both compared the findings of the MDT assessment and that of lumbar discography.[50, 82] I discussed these studies in Chapter 10 as they lend strong support to the intervertebral disc, with its reversible and directional nuclear location characteristics, being the underlying source of pain not only in patients with a directional preference, but in patients categorized as irreversible or irreducible derangements. To show that nuclear movement and fissure filling and emptying that occur with the performance of directional exercises or end-range positioning correlates with pain centralization and peripheralization would be a major contribution to understanding the biomechanical pathophysiology of the symptomatic intervertebral disc.

3. With the radiating or central LBP so often centralizing and abolishing, often from just a few repetitions of the appropriate direction of end-range testing and exercise, how would the positive findings of other evaluations be affected by such a rapid improvement in symptoms? Would a positive EMG, MRI, or discography findings done prior to the patient centralizing their pain be just as rapidly altered and improved, even reverting back to normal, as a result of the patient rapidly centralizing and abolishing their pain?

4. Our understanding and management of certain other LBP disorders will no doubt be influenced when the findings of the MDT assessment are reported for these more specific disorders. Looking for directional preference and centralization may uncover some new insights into these conventional diagnostic groups.

    a. Spondylolisthesis. Should they always avoid extending their lumbar spines, as conventional wisdom has us believe? Most MDT clinicians have noted that the pain of many patients labeled as having a "spondy" often have an extension directional preference, which means their pain centralizes, abolishes and then is usually also prevented using end-range lumbar *extension* tests and exercises. But how can that be when we have been taught for so long to not extend these patients and that their condition was likely even a result of extension trauma? One provocative study treated chronic patients with anterior spondys, retro- or posterior spondys, and no spondys with either flexion or extension oriented care consisting of directional exercises and bracing. To the surprise of the investigators, in all three radiographic groups, patients had much better outcomes with the extension treatment than with the flexion.[135] In their attempt to explain why all three radiographic subgroups did so well with extension, the investigators speculated that perhaps their pain had nothing to do with their radiographic findings but their common pain generator was an intervertebral disc that benefited from an extension program.

    Consequently, should these patients, just because they have this radiographic finding, be exempt from the same causes of LBP that afflict such a high percentage who have no radiographic changes and such a high prevalence for centralization with extension? After all, if spondylolisthesis is so often asymptomatic, then why can't it remain so in someone who develops LBP, perhaps non-specific LBP, and simply be an incidental x-ray finding?

This spondy subgroup that responds so well to extension is actually quite common in the experience of MDT clinicians but has yet to be reported in the scientific literature, even in the form of a case series. Given the provocative nature of this potential finding, it would seem that this study is likely to be done sooner rather than later. Confirmation of MDT clinicians' clinical experience would stimulate further disease process research. Thoughtful clinicians should also entertain the likelihood that undetected centralizers with spondys are also undergoing unnecessary surgery for recalcitrant pain attributed to their x-ray finding. The extent to which patients with rapidly reversible LBP are undergoing unnecessary surgery can easily be determined by collecting cohort data on how many pre-surgical spondys are found to be centralizers when provided the opportunity to be examined by a well-trained MDT clinician.

b. Spinal stenosis and pseudo-claudication symptoms. There are no published data here yet either, but it is not unusual for certain of these patients to substantially improve their walking tolerance after performing repeated end-range *extension* exercises. One could say that this subgroup has a paradoxical directional preference for extension, despite their history of experiencing less pain with forward bending and more when erect. So there seems to be two different directional subgroups, one that benefits surprisingly from performing end-range lumbar extension and the other from flexion.

5. How many patients treated with manipulation by their chiropractor, therapist, or osteopath are actually undetected centralizers who could recover using directed self-care while becoming independent of the health care system rather than risk becoming dependant on passive manual care and repeat visits to their provider? These patients are undergoing repeated manipulations unnecessarily, not unlike so many who take unneeded medications or undergo unnecessary MRIs, injections, and surgery.

Here is another opportunity for collaborative research with proponents of the Delitto classification system because they have identified criteria by which patients with acute LBP who can benefit from spinal manipulation can be identified.[28] But how many classified as manipulation candidates remain undetected centralizers due to the abbreviated examination in search of centralization who could do well with direction exercises and self-care rather than expose themselves to the risk of dependence on manual care?

I will discuss spinal manipulation further in Chapter 12 for it is not only an important topic relative to MDT, it is actually part of MDT care.

6. Many patients are currently being treated with "lumbar stabilization" exercise programs without the opportunity to undergo any directional preference assessment. How many LBP sufferers are being unnecessarily trained to maintain their lumbar spines in mid-range positions with no awareness that the very pain that is disrupting their lives can be eradicated and even prevented with repeated end-range exercises?

7. No cost-effectiveness studies have been conducted as yet into the use of MDT assessment to determine the economic value of identifying reversible (directional preference) subgroups. These are certainly relevant studies although some might hold that they may not be necessary when such an inexpensive intervention as MDT delivers such effective treatment in patients who otherwise would be subjected to multiple, expensive diagnostic and invasive interventions.

8. Further research is needed to document the prevalence of centralization and directional preference in patients who have reached the point of candidacy for lumbar surgery for pain. How can we justify performing surgery without knowing whether or not the patient has a directional preference that would typically lead to rapid reversal without surgery? Once again, this line of research will not be popular initially with some spine surgeons, and certainly not with the for-profit spinal instrumentation and high-tech companies, yet no surgeon and no such company would or should be comfortable with performing surgery on patients who can recover without surgery.

9. As discussed in Chapter 8, outcome prediction is such an important topic, demonstrated by the strong attention afforded psychosocial factors (yellow flags) in clinical guidelines and their perceived role as obstacles to recovery. There is some strong evidence however in support of centralization and directional preference as green flags with two studies providing evidence of the relative strength of these green flags and their absence (non-centralization) in comparison to the presence or absence of yellow flags.[68, 157] When common baseline psychosocial factors were compared with these pain response findings, the yellow flags were found to be non-predictors in the regression analysis compared with pain response findings.

Comparative predictive studies like this need repeating to better identify the relative strengths of baseline variables.

Interestingly, a multinational cohort study was conceived in 2003 to exhaustively evaluate the relative roles of baseline variables as outcome predictors. Many were polled to determine which potentially predictive factors should be included in the study. I made the case for including the MDT evaluation to determine the presence or absence of centralization and provided much of the evidence summarized in this book as support for the importance of centralization and directional preference as strong outcome predictors. Unfortunately, this information was not heeded and it was decided to omit these physical findings as part of the final design. Once again, the proverbial elephant in the room was ignored. Meanwhile, persisting funding shortcomings are likely to become insurmountable obstacles in that study.

More prognostic studies are needed to determine if excluding pain response findings is the only way that psychosocial factors become poor outcome predictors. At some point, other studies will investigate whether yellow flags tend to disappear as predictors of poor recovery in the presence of pain response findings as predictors.

Meanwhile, a systematic review of centralization prevalence, reliability in its identification, and prognostic studies was published in 2004[4] summarizing the many studies available at that time. This review concluded that "Centralization appears to identify a substantial subgroup of spinal patients; it is a clinical phenomenon that can be reliably detected, and is associated with a good prognosis. Centralization should be monitored in the examination of spinal patients."

10. In keeping with the theme of investigating the dynamics of recoveries rather than focusing only on obstacles for those who do not recover, the psychosocial benefits of empowering patients to be able to centralize and abolish their own LBP, especially chronic patients, should be studied. Anecdotal evidence suggests that the positive effects of this empowerment are substantial and very important from a psychosocial perspective.

Beyond simply measuring changes in depression, fear-avoidance, and somatization scales before and after successful treatment in directional preference patients, some of which is already reported,[90, 157] future studies might investigate changes in patients' locus of control related to their rather sudden empowerment once they learn that they can centralize and eliminate their own low back and leg pain. Once again, the high prevalence of this directional preference subgroup increases the importance of such studies.

The determination of these pain response and directional preference subgroups as baseline data will become a compelling piece of an increasing number of clinical research projects. This of course requires an appropriately trained clinician to provide this assessment as part of such a study. Fortunately, such clinicians are increasingly available to most research settings internationally. Identifying them is discussed in Chapter 13.

Funding sources

With funding so limited yet so critical for all health care research, agencies must allocate their resources wisely. Spending can be wisely guided for agencies that are aware of the value of LBP subgroup-based research in general, the A–D–T–O template specifically, along with the many research areas I've been presenting throughout this book.

It must again be emphasized, in light of the significant limitations inherent in conducting black box RCTs, there's little benefit in continuing to fund such studies. While there is always need to improve on the overall quality of how RCTs are conducted,[78] adopting the A–D–T–O strategic research model should be the strongest of priorities and the predominant guide for funding LBP clinical research at this time. Specifically, funding preference should initially be given to studies that address the Assessment–Diagnosis and Diagnosis–Treatment links before investing in far more expensive RCTs. Most currently used LBP treatments have yet to even establish which patients they can and can't successfully treat. For clinicians and researchers with an interest in investigating those treatments, establishing reliability in the assessment methods becomes the priority and funding should first focus on research targeting that Assessment–Diagnosis link until it is established or the assessment methods in question proven unreliable.

Guideline panels and MDT: at odds or consistent?

Presuming that all former guideline panels fundamentally possessed extensive knowledge of the LBP research literature, most recent international guideline panels seem committed more to being consistent and in agreement with prior guidelines than to stepping forward to review and consider previously overlooked non-RCT literature. The latter would surely shed light on what many of these same individuals have stated previously to be the most important and fundamental research priority in LBP: subgroup identification and validation.

One of the primary recommendations of LBP clinical guidelines has been to reassure individuals that their symptoms will most likely recover and therefore, barring symptoms and signs of "red flag" pathology, there's no need to undergo either expensive diagnostic or therapeutic interventions unless their symptoms persist for some designated period of time (six weeks is often used).

Consistent with that recommendation, when MDT assessment so commonly reveals the mechanical means by which patients can control and even eliminate their own pain, often rather quickly, as documented in the Long et al RCT, there is no more reassuring an experience for patients than to learn how to eliminate their own pain easily and quickly enabling them to return to or maintain their activities without aggravating their pain.

In addition to providing the ultimate in patient reassurance for so many, MDT emphasizes and teaches both patient self-care and the early return to activity and exercise, entirely consistent with current guideline recommendations.

It is interesting to note however that the first acute LBP guidelines didn't appear until the mid-'90s in the form of the U.S. Agency for Health Care Policy and Research guidelines.[10] McKenzie's first textbook however, that taught and advocated all these same guideline treatment principles was published in 1981, fourteen years before we had any guidelines at all.[101] Not only was McKenzie that far ahead of all clinical guidelines, but his observations and methods dramatically exceeded even today's best guidelines by teaching how to identify the means of providing *patient-specific,* rather than one-size-fits-all, self-care, which is the extent to which the most modern of clinical guidelines help us today.

So it is clear and important to note that self-care treatment methods of MDT were not developed *in response to* LBP clinical guideline recommendations but *preceded* them by 15–25 years. What remains a mystery today is how and why McKenzie's work, which so aligns itself with guideline recommendations, has been available for 25 years yet has managed to be overlooked, misunderstood, and just ignored by so many LBP experts who are expected, even mandated, as guideline panelists to be familiar with the LBP literature and the various methodologies for managing it, especially the more commonly used ones.

To date, the Danish clinical LBP guideline is the only one that acknowledges that McKenzie care is anything but extension exercises.[97] And I know from personal communication that they have been criticized by leaders of other European guidelines for recognizing the strength and validity of the science investigating the assessment process and the predictive quality of centralization.[96]

It is hard to argue with Spratt's statement that black box RCTs "will continue to be frustrating, meaningless, and even misleading."[133] Nevertheless, guideline panels continue to ignore the importance of reviewing those other study designs that identify LBP subgroups, specifically the importance of reliability and prospective cohort studies, while persisting with their current focus on black box RCTs. In that way, they far more resemble part of the problem than the solution. Claiming to be leaders in the solution of the LBP dilemma is what justifies government and other agencies and foundations to fund their work. Alternatively, by simply following the lead of so many who have stated the importance of focusing on subgroup-related studies,[14, 15, 36, 132, 133] guideline panels can greatly stimulate our rate of progress in understanding and managing LBP.

Let me also acknowledge that I am writing as an outsider to, and therefore merely an observer of, the guideline process. I have never been invited to be a member of any guideline panel or committee. I only know of one individual with any MDT expertise who served on such a panel and he states that his persistent efforts to present the evidence about MDT assessment, centralization and directional preference fell on deaf ears, was essentially ignored and was finally excluded from their guideline. He was unsuccessful in influencing the panel to refrain from adopting the scientifically unsupported "diagnostic triage" as the initial means of initial LBP classification.

So try as they may to portray objectivity and thoroughness in their literature reviews and methodologies, it seems apparent that guideline panels are strongly consensus-based and their membership selection is typically based on prior guideline experience and professional relationships. Such a selection process is essential to the perpetuation of consistent guidelines. But are consistent guidelines what serve the LBP population and its management best? We have certainly seen evidence of guideline deficiency being perpetuated by consensus in the European Acute LBP Clinical Guidelines where, again, we read: "A simple and practical classification, which has gained international acceptance, is by dividing acute low back pain into three categories—the so-called 'diagnostic triage.' "

Let me also add that, most panel members who, as individuals, advocate for certain clinical approaches, seem to have little understanding of the A–D–T–O research model and do not realize that validating their favorite clinical approach begins with reliability studies and not the conduct of one more black box RCT.

Just like clinicians, and all other human beings for that matter, scientists are not immune to tunnel vision and bias, and are naturally attracted to the comfort of their esteemed peers.

As I said in the Introduction, I am openly writing as an advocate for two stakeholder groups who are suffering from LBP, those who suffer unnecessarily with the physical symptoms and so often undergo unproven, ineffective non-operative care, as well as those caught up in paying the extraordinary cost of all this unnecessary care and disability. Perhaps these observations about the LBP guideline process will in some way be able to beneficially influence how future panels function.

PART 5
Considerations in
Mechanical Diagnosis & Therapy

Chapter 12
Mechanical Diagnosis & Therapy
and Manual Therapy

*"You cannot help men permanently by doing for them
what they could or should do for themselves."*
—*Abraham Lincoln*

The relationship between MDT and manual therapy is an important one because both are mechanical interventions directly applied to the spine to achieve symptomatic relief. Thus, their relationship, as well as the prominence of manual therapy use in low back care in general, is deserving of a separate chapter.

Background of manual therapy

Manual therapy is prominently used in the treatment of LBP by most chiropractors, and many physical therapists and osteopaths. Manual therapy applies external mechanical passive forces to the spine using the hands with the intent of providing symptomatic relief and functional improvement to those suffering with painful disorders of the spine.

Please note that my use of the term manual therapy is quite generic and I am not distinguishing amongst the wide array of manual interventions utilized by the many manual disciplines. No doubt many elitist manual practitioners are horrified that I would lump their skills with so many other disciplines.

The best known form of manual therapy is spinal *manipulation,* which provides a rapid (high-velocity) but small (low-amplitude) movement that is a thrust or push, applied directly to the joints between two adjacent vertebrae. The intent is to take these joints beyond their normal range of motion in the direction the force is applied. Notice, there's that word "direction" again.

A frequent objective is to achieve an audible joint sound, often attributed to cavitation, thought by most to be due to a release of gases under pressure from the posterior spinal facet joints. There is no evidence that achieving such a sound has any therapeutic value and there's even evidence to the contrary. Indeed, such joint sounds are routinely elicited even when asymptomatic individuals undergo spinal manipulation and therefore provide no insight into whether any benefit has been delivered to the pain-generating portion of the spine. It may be helpful to note that a frequently used term for manipulation by the chiropractic profession is "spinal adjustment."

Spinal *mobilization* is another commonly used manual technique that also moves the vertebral joints by bending the spine in a single direction, but applies the force slowly (low-velocity) and with progressively increasing distance. The intent is to stretch or move these same joints further than the individual themselves can move them.

An assortment of manual techniques is used that is often these clinicians' primary form of treatment. To my knowledge, there is little if any evidence linking the selection of such treatments to any reliable or validated assessment findings. The decision-making process regarding the selection of which manual techniques to use for any given patient is very elusive and hasn't yet been studied in anything resembling the A–D–T–O model. Such research would of course begin with reliability studies to determine subgroups that might benefit from some subgroup-specific form of manual therapy.

Applying passive end-range loading forces

When a mobilization or manipulation force is applied manually to the spine, the clinician typically bends or moves the spine passively in one direction, past its available end-range. Of course, passive end-range forces are also applied when patients perform repetitive end-range exercises as we've been describing within the MDT paradigm.

Manual therapy and repetitive end-range exercises as used in MDT are actually just two different ways of applying passive, single-direction end-range loading to the spine. The important difference between these two interventions is that manual therapy enables the clinician to apply a greater force to the spine than patients can apply to themselves through end-range exercises. A similar but lesser end-range directional force can be applied by patients themselves using exercises that can also be applied repetitively.

But how does a clinician know in what direction manual force should be applied? Outside the MDT assessment, it is difficult to get a consistent or principle-based answer to that question from manual clinicians. Again, I'm unaware of any evidence that matches any *reliable* clinical exam finding with any manual technique to demonstrate increased efficacy.

This is where the MDT *assessment* has considerable value. Both manual mobilization and patient-generated end-range movements also serve as tests when applied while monitoring for the pain response, specifically centralization. As we've been discussing, centralization indicates the underlying pain generator is rapidly reversible, whether that response is elicited using the MDT end-range loading tests or some form of manual force.

Thus, the clear similarity between MDT exercises and manual therapy is that they are both techniques that apply directional end-range loading forces to a symptomatic spine. In the case of MDT however, the symptomatic response then guides decision-making in the selection of beneficial treatment.

Manual therapy within Mechanical Diagnosis & Therapy (McKenzie care)

Unknown to many, manual therapy has an important and distinct role *within* the MDT paradigm of care. Manual therapy is in fact part of the formal education of MDT clinicians.

The key here is that not every patient with a reversible underlying pain source can apply sufficient end-range force to fully reverse it, that is, fully centralize or abolish the symptoms. Some reversible pain sources simply require more end-range force in the proper direction than the patient can provide themselves with repetitive end-range exercises. Although it is always more desirable to find a way for patients to do it all themselves, if progress is slow or has stopped in terms of acquiring full centralization, the brief use of manual mobilization in that same direction is often worthwhile.

It's helpful here to think of the repeated exercises performed within the MDT assessment as a form of spinal self-mobilization. The end-range force is just applied repetitively rather than with the extra force supplied by the manual clinician. We should also note that, although individuals are limited as far as the amount of force they can apply to their own spines,

"Not every patient with a reversible underlying pain source can apply sufficient end-range force to fully reverse it"

they have their own means of increasing the effectiveness of that force.

One technique for adding more force is to incorporate gravity. This is an important feature of the "press-up" technique (see Figure 7–2) by letting the patient's lumbar area maximally sag, assisted by gravity. Secondly, perhaps the most important way to be effective is to apply that end-range force repetitively. Some patients require more repetitions than others to maximize their beneficial pain response or to eliminate their pain. How many repetitions are needed is of course guided by the pain response.

In addition to gravity and repetition, a third useful factor is the frequency with which patients can apply these end-range forces. Unlike manual therapy, they are not restricted in applying this repetitive end-range force until their return appointment with their chiropractor or manual therapist. They can apply these forces many times a day, at home, at work, or, perhaps most importantly, whenever needed. The benefits of self-mobilization in terms of increased frequency and the timeliness of exercising relative to symptom behavior is a huge advantage in achieving long-term benefit with MDT compared with the short-term benefit attributed to manually applying the extra force during an office visit.

The ability and availability to apply these forces repetitively several times during the day likely explains why so many recover so quickly on their own, and then remain better. Although there are no data available yet to support this, there is little doubt amongst clinicians first trained in manual therapy who have then learned and now use MDT methods that many patients who they previously felt required manual mobilization or manipulation can just as easily learn to do it all themselves. These practitioners see their patients recover more quickly, but just as important, these patients are able to maintain that improvement long term, with most having no need to return for further care.

Although more data is needed, the nearly universal observations of MDT clinicians are that only a relatively small percentage of patients with a directional preference are unable to generate sufficient end-range force to centralize or abolish their own pain. But it is this small subgroup, and only this small subgroup, where manual testing, while monitoring the immediate pain response, is helpful in initiating or progressing centralization toward recovery.

I said "only this small subgroup" should have manual testing because those who are progressing nicely with self-generated forces (exercises) should not be introduced to manual interventions, given the risks involved in doing so, which I will explain shortly. This reasoning is analogous to not introducing surgery to patients who are progressing nicely without it.

I would add one more very important point. Whenever manual therapy is required to begin the reversal/centralization process, it is usually only needed on one or maybe two occasions. Once the reversal of the underlying lesion begins, that is, the pain has started to centralize, the patient can usually be taught how to then maintain and improve that centralization by performing a directional exercise.

In these cases, the role of manual therapy within the MDT paradigm is simple: *to restore to the patient their ability to self-treat.* With self-treatment being the objective, manual therapy's role then becomes much better defined and appreciated.

Manual therapy's risks and contraindications

Although there are reported cases of manipulation forces actually causing further spinal injury,[124] such complications are exceedingly rare. A much more common complication of manual therapy is the dependence upon it that patients develop. Whenever short-term improvement occurs related to any intervention, whenever those symptoms return again, most patients tend to return to that intervention for further assistance.

We've already discussed the high recurrence rate of LBP episodes. But even within a single episode, dependency becomes an issue with short-term relief interventions, whether it is to medication, manual therapy, or some other passive intervention.

Most clinicians would agree that one of the most important objectives of any medical treatment should be to empower patients to be self-sufficient. If there is a way for patients to take responsibility for their own health, in this case through effective and patient-specific self-treatment of their LBP, then manual therapy has the potential to become an obstacle to achieving self-sufficiency.

Just as any other form of passive care that provides short-term pain relief, manual therapy risks teaching patients to become dependant on their manual treatment and hence upon their manual clinician. Their "experiential" education, coupled with the explicit advice provided by their clinician, teaches them to come back for more treatment whenever their pain returns. Manual therapy, in and of itself, teaches them that, to get rid of their own pain, they must return to their practitioner. If the pain returns, their thinking is that they obviously need further manual therapy.

Although the frequency of such cases is not well documented, some manual therapy clinicians intentionally promote such dependency for their own benefit rather than that of the patient. Another treatment strategy, often interpreted as a marketing ploy, is "preventive" manual care of asymptomatic children. Such clinicians would view dependency as good for business, while advocating it as good for their patients, but without a shred of evidence of benefit. Some clinicians are quite good at nurturing a most unfortunate web of dependant thinking and care.

However, the great majority of manual clinicians are very sincere about providing quality care for their patients. Many perhaps simply don't understand or don't know how to avoid the negative long-term consequences of their manual care. Most also have no understanding of how easily and commonly patients can reverse their own low back disorder.

In contrast, MDT gives patients the opportunity to learn how to monitor their own symptom response to their own positions, movements, and exercises, and to exercise and modify positions as needed to centralize, eliminate, and prevent their own symptoms. It is this form of experiential education that is so empowering and so valuable. It is this same education that manual clinicians deprive their patients by moving too quickly to manual techniques without first exploring, and I should say without exhausting, the possibilities that there is a means by which the patient can centralize, abolish, and prevent their own symptoms.

Many manual therapists and chiropractors, endeared to the use of manual techniques, justify manipulating nearly everyone in a one-size-fits-all philosophy of care. In actuality however, only a very few patients are unable to generate sufficient force on their own, thereby needing some brief manual intervention. Robin McKenzie, who you'll recall started his career as a manual therapist, has many times said that we cannot go on manipulating everyone in order to deliver the benefit to the very few who really need it. He has always contended that, if it is possible to teach a patient exercises that allow him to manage his own problem, manual interventions should be avoided. Further, every such patient should be provided with self-care education and every clinician should be obliged to supply it.

Thus, once again, patient selection becomes the key. The manual spine professions, by not embracing patients' common ability to successfully self-treat, will continue to contribute to, and encourage, dependency on themselves while unnecessarily increasing health care costs. Spine care clinicians of all types, whether manual clinicians, medication prescribers, injectionists, or surgeons, need to learn who can and can't self-treat with end-range repetitive exercises; i.e., who does and does not have a reversible underlying pain source that will respond to simple repetitive end-range loading exercises. Their favorite interventions are valuable in those patients who cannot successfully self-treat but are otherwise unnecessary and significant drivers of high costs for most individuals with LBP.

A growing number of the chiropractic, osteopathic and physical therapy manual groups are recognizing and acknowledging the risk of creating dependency in their patients when they are only able to deliver a short-term benefit with their manual therapy techniques. It is an understandable challenge for them to refrain from using their hands in order to fully exhaust patients' ability to eliminate their own pain with end-range repetitive exercises. This is analogous to the challenge for surgeons to exhaust all non-surgical options prior to operating. It is the mantra we speak, but how often and thoroughly do we do as we say?

Thus, both repetitive end-range exercises and manual therapy have their own strengths, benefits and limitations within the MDT paradigm. But the overriding goal of MDT, or any other form of care for that matter, is to move patients toward achieving independence in dealing with both their current and any future symptoms. Alternatively, manual therapy engenders dependence on the clinician's skills, including teaching patients to return for more manual therapy for any future problems.

Summary

Manual therapy is a valuable intervention but it is only necessary in a small subset of the very large directional preference subgroup. It is currently greatly overused in low back care, causing unnecessary dependency on the clinician's skills. But once you appreciate that its primary role should be to restore patients' abilities to self-treat, then it becomes clear that only a small group needs manual therapy to effect positive change.

Manual therapy plays an important role for the patient with a reversible problem who cannot self-generate enough end-range force to commence that reversal process hallmarked by pain centralization. Manual therapy can help get things started by applying an extra external force. In light of the important objective of teaching patients self-sufficiency, manual therapy should only be used if self-generated forces have been exhausted, and then it is usually only needed once or twice. Manual therapy is simply not necessary in the majority of LBP patients due to the ability of their underlying pain generator to respond so well to self-generated repetitive end-range directional loading.

This chapter began with a quote from Abraham Lincoln: "You cannot help men permanently by doing for them what they could or should do for themselves." This is of course particularly relevant to clinicians who provide manual therapy as their primary spinal treatment. On a similar line of thought, Thomas Szacz offered this sound advice to patients regarding manual care: "Don't bite the hand that feeds you unless it is keeping you from feeding yourself."

Chapter 13

Mechanical Diagnosis & Therapy and Credentialing

A thorough MDT assessment enables the identification of pain patterns patients are exhibiting and then teaching self-care principles and individualized instructions. This whole process often takes 20–30 minutes or even longer in more complex patients. With the average length of primary care office visits now only 8–10 minutes, there is insufficient time for most physicians to assess, educate, and initiate low back self-care, even if the physician were motivated to invest the necessary time and money to be properly educated in conducting this form of care.

Nevertheless, the critical questions that must be asked when seeing each new LBP patient remain: is this patient's problem rapidly reversible or not? Can the pain be centralized and abolished? And does the low back problem have a directional preference? If the answers to these questions are "yes," then recoveries are usually rapid and confident and the time and money saved can be substantial. Time and money are saved with such a focused assessment by:

1. the patients, who so often get prompt answers as well as the ultimate in reassurance of recovery by experiencing their pain centralizing and abolishing. Subsequent visits are few in number so time away from work for appointments and cost of travel is minimized.
2. the payers, since the cost of a single or a few visits is substantially less than the costs associated with many visits, and expensive but unnecessary diagnostic tests and treatments are avoided; and
3. the clinicians, who can spend their clinical time on those patients in need of their care where known efficacious therapies are not yet well established.

The cost of such an assessment is so minor compared with the immense potential expense of non-recovery. As the Fram oil filter ad said: "You can pay me now [a small amount for an oil change] or pay me later [a large amount to replace a ruined engine]."

Three published surveys have documented the apparent widespread use of the MDT approach to spinal pain, both within and outside the U.S.[9, 60, 86] But how well trained are all those clinicians who claim to be using these methods?

It is logical that more and better training in delivering any skill would create higher quality in its delivery and, as a consequence, in achieving successful outcomes. To date, only those clinicians that have attained the McKenzie Institute Credentialed or Diplomaed recognition have been shown to be reliable in their interpretation of the assessment and in determining patient classifications (see Chapter 8).

In twenty years of referring LBP patients for MDT, my experience has overwhelmingly been that patients were far more likely to have successful recoveries when referred to someone with these specific credentials. *The chances of missing a centralizer with a good prognosis were much greater if I referred patients to a practitioner who was not at least MDT credentialed.*

So what is all this credentialing stuff? It's an important question with an important answer, not only for physicians who wish to refer patients for this assessment, but for researchers who wish to incorporate this assessment within the context of a research project.

The educational and credentialing process

Whether you are a clinician, researcher, patient, or payer, it is vital to have some understanding of the substantial educational and credentialing process clinicians complete to become credentialed or receive their Diploma in MDT.

The McKenzie Institute International, www.mckenziemdt.org[127], is a non-profit, educational organization that conducts four sequential MDT courses in more than thirty countries. These are post-graduate courses 3–4 days in length with participants encouraged to space them at least several months apart to provide themselves with ample time for clinical utilization of the methods before progressing to the next course. It is common for clinicians to complete these four courses over 18–24 months. There is now a fifth course that focuses on the use of MDT assessment methods for painful disorders in the extremities.

The satisfactory completion of these courses qualifies one to take the MDT Credentialing exam, a rigorous one-day evaluation using paper-pencil, video, and actors serving as patients to evaluate candidates' clinical assessment and treatment skills. Successfully completing this exam signifies competency, but what the McKenzie Institute states is at a minimal or the lowest level of competency in delivering reliable MDT assessment and treatment. The reliability data would so far bear this out.

Each U.S. credentialed practitioner must then participate in specific continuing educational activities during each three year period to remain on the MDT Clinician Referral database. Other countries have similar educational opportunities to enable Credentialed clinicians to maintain their high level of competency.

Having passed the Credentialing exam, competency can be elevated further since practitioners are then qualified to engage the MDT Diploma course that consists of nine full-time weeks of a clinical tutorial; i.e., a mentorship, as well as 360 hours focused on clinical reasoning, problem-solving, conditions suitable and unsuitable for MDT treatment, and learning critical analysis of the scientific literature. This culminates with a Diploma Final Examination.

The McKenzie Institute faculty members, who now reside in 25 different countries, teach the four basic MDT courses. They must be a Diplomate and have completed an extensive two-year probationary faculty training program as well as be engaged in a minimum of 500 hours of on-going clinical work annually to continue teaching. These standards and rigorous requirements illustrate the high clinical and educational quality of these experts in the field.

The network of available clinicians

Within the U.S., there are currently more than 1,700 Credentialed MDT clinicians, mostly physical therapists, but this includes a growing number of chiropractors and a handful of MDs. Currently there are also 110 MDT Diplomates in the U.S.A. and over 400 MDT Diplomates around the world.

This network of McKenzie/MDT specialists has been steadily growing for many years. This growth and this entire educational system is a unique international phenomenon. It is especially impressive given the huge effort and expense required of each clinician to attain these levels of expertise and, perhaps most importantly, given the lack of any significant financial incentive to do so. At this point in time, there is virtually no financial recognition of their skills or clinical value. Their greatest incentive is the appreciation and satisfaction this paradigm offers them in making objective clinical decisions using the reliable assessment and classification process they have learned that guides their clinical decision-making in determining validated patient-specific self-care.

Hopefully there will at some point be some financial recognition for the skills and value these clinicians bring to low back care. The availability of this paradigm would increase immensely if some financial incentive to become trained was available.

So who *really* knows MDT?

In today's competitive health care marketplace, it is common for physical therapists and chiropractors *to claim* to know McKenzie care, regardless of their level of education. I've heard such claims *to know it* from those who had only attended a single in-service in their clinic led by someone who had only attended the introductory course.

Suffice it to say, in seeking someone to adequately deliver the MDT product, the patient, referring physician, and even the payer would be wise to first determine whether the clinician has passed the Credentialing or Diploma examination. You are especially fortunate to have access to someone with an MDT Diploma.

As I said earlier, I have had many different MDT educational levels represented in the therapists and chiropractors to whom I have referred my patients over the years. In nearly every case, there is a substantial difference in the success of my patients' recoveries by those who are Credentialed or Diplomaed and those who were not.

You will surely find, as I did, that, due to the frequency with which MDT is requested, clinicians not fully trained, including some with the smallest of introductions to it, often claim "to know McKenzie" or be "McKenzie-trained." Therefore, when searching for someone well trained, I recommend calling offices and clinics to inquire whether they have someone who has passed either the McKenzie credentialing or diploma exams. Assistance in locating such an individual is also available by going to the McKenzie Institute website (www.mckenziemdt.org) where a current directory is available. If no such person is available in your geographic area of interest, the next best thing is to inquire locally as to who has progressed the furthest through the four basic McKenzie courses described earlier.

MDT reliability tied to educational level: a validation of MDT Credentialing?

The reliability of implementing the MDT assessment and classification system has thus far been reported to be high in studies where Credentialed MDT practitioners performed the assessments. The prevalence of centralization and directional preference reported in these studies has been 70% or higher in acute LBP patients and hovering around 50% in those with chronic LBP (see Chapter 8). In contrast, far lower prevalence (29%) has been reported in studies where unqualified or minimally-trained clinicians performed the testing in search of centralization.[17]

Given the very high recovery rates of centralizing patients when treated with exercises and posture interventions consistent with their directional preference, there is a very high cost associated with mis-classifying a centralizer, which so far appears to be quite common when centralization assessments are performed by non-MDT-Credentialed clinicians.

Physician education in MDT

Most physicians, faced with the brevity of time to spend with each new patient, including those with complex low back problems, are reluctant to spend the time required to properly conduct a reliable MDT assessment. Most establish a relationship with one or more physical therapists or chiropractors in their communities who can provide a thorough rendition of this assessment and refer their patients for what often becomes an extension of their own initial evaluation. Close and very rewarding working relationships are established between physicians and these MDT practitioners, working together as a team to address the low back needs of these patients.

It is interesting to watch as physicians are looking for well-trained MDT practitioners to work with just as there are MDT practitioners searching for physicians with an understanding and appreciation for MDT care.

To that end, it is unnecessary for a physician who will refer to Credentialed MDT practitioners to become fully trained in MDT themselves, however it is very helpful for the welfare of his or her patients to have a good overview of MDT that provides a solid understanding and appreciation for it.

Recognizing that many physicians would not invest even four days to attend the initial McKenzie Institute lumbar course, an alternative educational opportunity that has provided an excellent introduction to McKenzie care is a one- or two-day overview course I have co-taught periodically over the past 18 years with one of the McKenzie Institute faculty members. It has always been received with enthusiasm by those who attended, but the challenge has always been to attract enough attendees to financially support it given the low level of awareness of the value of McKenzie care amongst so many medical disciplines. It remains a viable physician education tool should the awareness of the value of McKenzie care grow sufficiently to support it. Although this book serves similar value, there are many aspects of the MDT clinical system that are normally part of the course that simply cannot be covered as effectively within this book.

PART 6
Improving Low Back Pain Outcomes and Reducing Costs Sooner Rather Than Later

Chapter 14
How Long Does Change Take?

In his book entitled *Diffusion of Innovation*, Everett Rogers describes the typical pace and pattern with which most new innovations are adopted into general use.[118] Due to many factors, widespread adoption does not typically occur quickly.

He points out that a new innovation is first adopted by a small group of risk-taking "innovators" (see Figure 14–1). It is their acceptance of, and enthusiasm for, the new innovation that then stimulates others to also adopt. He calls this second group "Early Adopters." They are followed by the "Early Majority," then the "Late Majority," and finally by the "Laggards," the last group to come on board. Skepticism and tradition-bound thinking characterize both the Late Majority and Laggards.

This same diffusion pattern depicts what has been happening in the adoption of MDT low back care around the world. The "Innovator" group, obviously led by Robin McKenzie, includes those low back clinicians who became convinced of the merits of this approach back in the late '70s and throughout the '80s. It was clinicians' clinical results as they utilized these methods that motivated them to further adopt and persist in using these methods of care. In the past 15–20 years, a worldwide cadre of "Early Adopters" in turn has learned, and now utilizes, promotes, and teaches these methods.

As we see in Figure 14–1, this Early Adopter group is quite small compared with the wide spectrum of back care practitioners, most of whom still remain either unfamiliar with, or misinformed about, this MDT paradigm of care. This includes a sizable group that has had some exposure to MDT, and can therefore claim familiarity with it, but is not using it effectively due to their inadequate training (see Chapter 13).

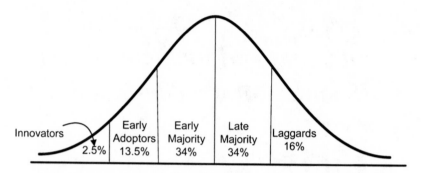

Figure 14–1: Rogers's adopter categories for innovations.

It is likely that the Laggards will include those strongly vested in other clinical paradigms, in flawed beliefs about the nature of LBP, or who currently view McKenzie clinicians as cult members. I should note however that there have been some noteworthy individuals who in the past have been hard-core opponents of MDT who over time recognized the evidence and the successful outcomes of patients so treated.

The extensive spread of MDT to more than 30 countries to date has actually been quite remarkable considering it was based primarily on "word-of-mouth" recommendation by satisfied patients and clinicians. The emerging literature support over the past 15 years, in my opinion, has actually had only a minor effect on this growth, related to a general lack of MDT acknowledgment amongst the research leaders and guideline communities.

At the present pace of adoption, one might estimate from Rogers's template that it may be another 30 years before MDT is adopted by even the "Early Majority." However, one could also foresee the rate of this adoption increasing significantly as the existing A–D–T–O evidence becomes more widely known across the full spectrum of LBP stakeholders and as additional studies emerge in the next five years. Based on the large body of current evidence that so clearly reinforces the positive clinical experience of thousands of MDT trained clinicians worldwide over these past 25 years, it is my personal expectation and prediction that future studies will not only reinforce the findings of existing studies but will greatly add to our understanding of LBP mechanisms and anatomic sources as they focus more on this large green flag subgroup of centralization/directional preference patients.

Can future savings in low back care occur sooner rather than later?

You have hopefully read enough to understand the strength of the MDT-targeted research. More RCTs will no doubt follow, but there is little reason to believe that, as long as MDT is accurately and fully implemented, their outcomes will be substantially different from the many cohorts and several subgroup-focused RCTs that have already been published. They are just too consistently good and too numerous. As I said earlier, there is no longer need for more reliability studies to serve as proof on concept, even though there will always be a need to determine that the reliability of various clinical and research groups is established and maintained.

There is also no question about the strong green flag predictive power of centralization and directional preference. The high centralization and directional preference prevalence also seems well-established, at least when the exam is performed by Credentialed MDT practitioners.

So let's now consider the potential savings and improved quality of lives associated with some intentional efforts to speed-up this MDT adoption rate. At nearly $100 billion per year overhead in the U.S. alone, the cost-reduction over the next 25 years for more quickly implementing MDT on a widespread basis could easily climb into the hundreds of billions of dollars in the U.S. alone. Must this all take 25 years to develop?

Let's look at some strategies that can speed the adoption of this MDT paradigm.

Chapter 15

Strategies for Cutting Low Back Pain
Suffering and Spending

In this chapter, I want to share some thoughts in how we might build on all this MDT evidence with the intent to bring relief sooner to the millions struggling with LBP itself and for those who are experiencing the economic pain of paying for this huge problem.

Building on Rogers's diffusion of innovation model,[118] Greenalgh et al have described three mechanisms that influence the rate at which innovation spreads. They call them "letting it happen," "helping it happen," and "making it happen."[69] I'd even add a fourth influence, albeit a negative one: "keeping, or discouraging, it from happening" (see Figure 15–1). I'm going to touch on each of these influences of the spread of MDT and, more specifically, of the MDT assessment.

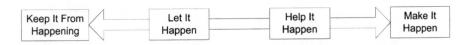

Figure 15–1: Influencing the spread of innovation.

Keeping it from happening

I have no data to support what I am about to tell you, just my personal encounters over the past 25 years with LBP clinicians of all disciplines, researchers, systematic reviewers, and guideline participants.

Over those years, there have clearly been influences that have slowed the spread of MDT care. Many detractors have consistently expressed a negative view of MDT. What is clear from their writings and from my many personal conversations and correspondence with systematic reviewers, guideline chairmen and panelists, is that they just don't understand that McKenzie care is anything more than extension exercises. Perhaps not independent from this fact is their apparent lack of regard for the MDT discipline in general. Consequently, their interest in learning more about MDT is often non-existent, or at least meager, to the point that it becomes a matter of concern when this involves national and international LBP leaders who are looked to as experts in determining the latest and best ways to manage LBP.

I had a conversation at an international spine conference with one of the world's best-known and respected LBP experts. When I brought up the topic of, and the evidence for, centralization, he acknowledged his unfamiliarity with that body of literature and his inability to comment. On one hand, I appreciated his honesty, that he didn't attempt to portray himself, like so many others, as knowledgeable when he wasn't. Yet, to this acclaimed LBP expert, one of the most thoroughly studied and validated clinical findings in the LBP literature (centralization) was and remains unknown with no sign of interest on his part to learn more.

It is understandable that many of you reading this book would not have previously known the LBP literature I've presented, especially when it has been overlooked in the LBP guidelines you've read. As you are well aware by now, that was one of my main reasons for writing *Rapidly Reversible Low Back Pain*. However, it is quite another thing for those mandated, even funded in many cases, as clinical guideline chairpersons and participants to be unaware that McKenzie care involves an assessment and classification system and is not just extension exercise treatment.

One interesting view of McKenzie care that has persisted in the some minds for many years is that McKenzie-trained clinicians comprise "a cult" led by their "guru." This even became public way back in 1986 at a large U.S. spine conference. As an audience member, I asked one of the speakers, a prominent international figure in LBP who was fielding questions from the audience after his presentation, for his view of centralization and McKenzie methods of care. His response was: "McKenzie is a preacher and I don't get mixed up in religious matters."

For a luminary to respond in this fashion no doubt influenced many in attendance that day. I believe that opinion has influenced others over the years, most importantly, many LBP leaders. It came to my attention again just a few months ago in a private discussion with another prominent low back clinician. As I began to draw attention to the many MDT-supportive studies, his somewhat agitated response included his view that the McKenzie approach was "a cult" and that many other LBP leaders felt that way. There was absolutely no interest on his part for an intellectual discussion of the published literature. How can we expect to make progress in our management and research of LBP with such mind sets prevalent amongst the leaders in the field?

Similarly, there have been spine clinicians over the years who have expressed discomfort that such a widely acclaimed paradigm as MDT was named after a person (i.e., "the cult leader") even though he is its developer. It was in part to address this specific negative bias that this approach was re-named "Mechanical Diagnosis and Therapy." While nearly all McKenzie-trained clinicians have the highest regard for Robin McKenzie and his clinical observations, their loyalty to, and enthusiasm for, his methods of care are unquestionably based on their own clinical results, their own patients' recoveries, and the literature that continues to scientifically validate their own clinical experience.

So make note that those who voice the greatest skepticism about MDT care, MDT-focused literature, and even about this book, may have a bias of their own that is as strong or stronger than the bias they so often assign to MDT clinicians enthusiastic about these methods of low back care. At the very least, these folks are unfamiliar with the MDT assessment and classification protocol and mistakenly view MDT care as consisting only of extension exercise treatment. Most are also largely, if not completely, reliant on black box RCTs. Paradoxically, many also assent to the importance of identifying LBP subgroups while overlooking the essential study designs required to accomplish that task; i.e., reliability and predictive cohorts we've discussed within the A–D–T–O clinical research model back in Chapter 6.

Some have raised other questions that may play a role with "keeping it from happening." What personal consequences would arise if an inexpensive solution for much of LBP were discovered and put into practice, especially if their expertise and hard work wasn't part of such a development? Some have wondered: if centralization and solving LBP was as simple as McKenzie followers claim it to be, certainly other LBP experts who for decades have devoted their clinical and research careers to searching for LBP "truth" would have found these same things long ago. There was a time early in his work that McKenzie thought those same things. He found out differently.

Others who hear and begin to think about, but still don't understand, directional preference express that it is nothing new. After all, we've known for a long time that LBP patients often worsen when they bend forward. Again, how much LBP research funding; i.e., researchers' livelihood, would disappear if the high costs of low back care were slashed by identifying effective subgroup-specific treatments for most with LBP?

There's one more thing. Like most other health care fields, LBP clinical care is top-heavy with high-priced specialists who routinely advocate their own patient-selection process and prescribe their own interventions, often lucrative ones, for their patients. This powerful influence from individual clinicians and their specialty societies becomes evident whenever the efficacy or appropriateness of their treatments is called into question.

Obviously, these views address three of the most common issues for all of mankind: ego, power, and money. But then, why would we expect it to be any different in the field of health care than in any other area of human endeavor?

On one hand, these are not comfortable things to present, yet they are highly relevant to the topic of this chapter. With them as background, it is easier to understand why the MDT paradigm of care, which has been fully described in textbooks for 25 years,[101, 103] in many review articles,[42-49, 53] taught in literally thousands of courses worldwide, and now quite thoroughly studied and supported by a growing body of scientific literature, continues to be ignored as a LBP assessment and classification system by so many LBP experts.

Letting it happen

The concept of "letting it happen" would imply the absence of any substantial, focused stimulus directed at an innovation with the intent of influencing its spread of adoption. Realistically however, "letting it happen" always involves a mix of positive and negative forces that influence both providers and consumers of health care. The "keeping it from happening" forces we just discussed might be construed by some as just a part of "letting it happen" since there will always be naysayers in any innovation process, with some of those likely ending up as Everett's "laggards" (Figure 14–1).

Alternatively, we must also acknowledge the influence of commonplace advocacy efforts by members of the various low back disciplines who promote their paradigm of care, often based simply on their own anecdotal experiences. My own efforts over the years in speaking and writing on behalf of MDT could be construed either as part of "letting it happen" or even "helping it happen." We'll get to more of that "helping it happen" in a minute.

But in the big picture, the spread of MDT utilization over the past 25 years is probably best interpreted as following the "letting it happen" pattern. Its impressive worldwide growth is just that much more remarkable since it seems fundamentally related to word-of-mouth endorsements from satisfied, often enthusiastic, patients and clinicians.

The enthusiasm of MDT-trained clinicians is unusually common, so much so as to sometimes draw attention either from those curious about such enthusiasm or from those who feel there must be some brainwashing going on.

I recall John Frymoyer's reaction to my growing interest and enthusiasm for the McKenzie approach to back care in the early '80s. A true pioneer and sage in spine care, Dr. Frymoyer was for many years the Chairman of the Department of Orthopedic Surgery at the University of Vermont in Burlington. It was in the late '70s and early '80s, when I was in private practice, first in Vermont and then just across Lake Champlain from Burlington, in northeast New York State, he watched me become increasingly interested in McKenzie care and was intrigued by my shifting interest toward treating low back pain non-operatively. Rather than dismissing me for this eccentricity, he instead invited me to present the McKenzie paradigm at his orthopedic grand rounds, stating that he had to find out more about anything that motivated an orthopedic surgeon to become enthused about the non-operative care of LBP. Unlike so many LBP leaders, he wanted to hear and learn more about this and bring it to the attention of his orthopedic colleagues and residents.

I mentioned earlier that it is very common for MDT practitioners when beginning to use these methods to state that, for the first time, they feel as though they have something to offer their patients that targets their actual back problem in a way that provides clear and lasting relief. Indeed, that was my own observation of the centralization phenomenon more than 25 years ago, followed closely by my realization that clinical decisions could be both individualized and objective. It was the ability to rapidly reverse someone's underlying low back condition that first caught my attention, that over time led to me to shift my professional focus away from sports medicine to non-operative spine care.

There are thousands of similar stories from clinicians around the world who attended their initial McKenzie Institute educational course. These courses featured live assessments of LBP patients never seen by the course instructor, and then treatment guidance and follow-up with each patient on each subsequent day of the course. Centralization occurs commonly in these patients, regardless of which of 25 or 30 countries is hosting the course.

It should also be noted that this extensive worldwide growth has happened despite two other influential negative forces: 1) a nearly complete absence of recognition by most international guidelines of the MDT assessment and, even more importantly, 2) the minimal, if any, financial incentive for clinicians to pursue the required training to provide this type of care. Let's explore this second point now.

Helping it happen

Given the substantial evidence supporting the widespread use of the MDT assessment, speeding the spread of this innovation seems both appropriate and important. The billions of dollars to be saved and the millions of lives whose quality can be improved justifies finding ways to accelerate the spread in utilization of this MDT assessment beyond just the "letting it happen" forces that have prevailed for the past 25 years.

"Helping it happen" is actually quite a common phenomenon in health care. Financial incentives immediately come to mind as a powerful force in the adoption of any new innovation or technology. This is no better illustrated in spine care than clinicians' aggressive pursuit of specialized training that enables them to provide a new and usually expensive innovation that is likewise financially rewarding to them. This is quite common in spine care. A conspicuous example a few years ago was the intense pursuit of education in how to perform intradiscal electrothermal therapy procedures (IDET) for treating symptomatic chronic degenerative lumbar disc disease. More recently, a similar rush for expensive training has taken place in how to implant artificial discs. I am told that twenty-five hundred U.S. spine surgeons completed this training within six months of the FDA approval of artificial disc arthroplasty at just one arthroplasty educational center, with 120 more trainees scheduled every week for the subsequent six months.

Coincidently, while writing this very section of the book, as a member of the North American Spine Society, I received an email soliciting me to join a new group called the Association of Ethical Spine Surgeons[120] whose purpose is to provide increased public awareness of the detrimental financial influence of the medical industry on many spine surgeons and their patients. Let it be known that NASS likewise clearly objects to such influences. This email then spoke of the "pervasive effect on the practice of medicine" on the part of a "small minority of spine surgeons (who) have become marketing men for big business," shamelessly promoting surgical products under the veil of clinical research. This form of "helping it happen" places the welfare of the industry and these surgeons far ahead of patients' welfare.

In Chapter 2, we discussed Dr. John Wennberg's position that by turning out so many spine surgeons who can provide these innovations, we are actually increasing the "supply side" forces in the spine care marketplace, which in turn naturally increases the number of these procedures offered and performed, as well as substantially raising the incomes of those providing these procedures.

Given the MDT data regarding lumbar disc surgical candidates however, we need to ask again: how many have already undergone, and every day are still undergoing, an IDET, disc arthroplasty procedure, fusion, or even routine disc herniation surgery for that matter, *unnecessarily*? Once centralization and directional preference are detected, patients usually experience a very satisfying, even excellent and often rapid, outcome if treated appropriately.

Another far more familiar means of "helping it happen" is the marketing of medications by pharmaceutical companies that uses "drug reps" to target doctors and national advertising to reach the public. Such marketing for analgesics, anti-inflammatories, and muscle relaxants for LBP are no exception, comprising the biggest single LBP expense.[141]

But now consider the uneven playing field relevant to the adoption of MDT care. First, MDT insurance reimbursement does not begin to recognize the significant post-graduate training time and expense required to acquire MDT skills nor the value of the reliable and valuable findings that this assessment provides to the clinical decision-making process for each patient. There is consequently little if any financial incentive to become trained nor is there the financial means for this group to lobby on their own behalf as is so routinely done by the much higher paid or larger groups of clinicians.

We must also consider the influence of clinical guidelines whose intent is to "help it happen;" "it" in this case being evidence-based low back care, as determined by carefully selected leaders in the field of LBP. Their primary objectives are to decrease the use of interventions with evidence of non-efficacy while encouraging the use of those with documented efficacy. However, as we discussed in the Tension Cycle in Chapter 3, their efforts through guideline recommendations to help it happen are undermined by clinicians' widespread non-compliance with those recommendations.

There are also administrative means intended to "help" influence the direction of patient care, such as requiring second opinions and pre-authorizations prior to more expensive procedures. Clinician profiling, or so-called "report cards," are a more recent strategy that tracks individual clinicians' low back care recommendations to determine the degree to which they comply, or don't comply, with clinical guidelines. Developers and advocates of these methodologies include the National Committee for Quality Assurance (NCQA)[107] and their esteemed spine experts who created NCQA's Spine Care Recognition Program whose stated intent is to "promote excellence in treating back pain." The program will identify and reward physicians and chiropractors who deliver currently recognized "high-quality, evidence-based care" by providing acute LBP patients with a clear understanding of appropriate treatment options as defined in recent guidelines. Keep in mind that, based on the content of current guidelines, such programs reward the use of one-size-fits-all, non-specific advice, and activity encouragement for acute LBP.

"Helping MDT happen" benefits all stakeholders

The good news I'm trying to convey is that promoting MDT is not just a win-win situation, it is win-win-win-win-win. Every LBP stakeholder stands to benefit in one way or another from implementing MDT on a wide scale. Let's review how each might benefit.

Patients: The data are clear. Most LBP patients have a directional preference and most can therefore learn to eliminate the pain of their current episode providing they are given the opportunity to be evaluated by an appropriately trained MDT clinician. In doing so, patients emerge empowered to recognize those mechanical factors which have been bringing on their prior episodes as well as how to prevent or quickly eliminate any future pain. This further enables them to have a far greater chance to become and remain independent of formal health care, rather than dependent on it for the care of their persisting or recurring low back disorder.

<u>Clinicians</u>: I guarantee that medical and surgical physicians, PTs, chiropractors, and osteopaths will have far greater satisfaction in their practices once they are able to objectively individualize their care using reliable, validated findings added to their current patient selection protocols.

The early and rapid recoveries possible with MDT have two important benefits that clinicians value: 1) pre-existing and secondary behavioral factors have far less opportunity to become operative; and 2) the underlying mechanical pathology has no opportunity to deteriorate further over time due to the obvious benefit it receives as it returns then to full and pain-free range of lumbar motion and activity.

This is excellent news for primary care physicians who are at the forefront of low back care, who are expected to provide relief for patients' persisting pain, both now and during their recurrences, appreciating that they often deteriorate over time, and well aware of the very real potential for developing medication dependency, especially opiates. This latter issue is a very real and common challenge. Providing pain relief for a mechanical problem using mechanical self-care interventions is so much more attractive and effective than dealing with the pressure of trying to manage mechanical pain using drugs.

While spine surgeons will understandably be concerned about MDT reducing their surgical volume and pain management their injection volumes, there will still be plenty of spine surgery and injections to do and it is difficult to put a price on the benefits and satisfaction for all parties at improving the patient selection process and avoiding an unnecessary surgical and injection procedures when centralization and pain abolition are elicited during an MDT assessment. Many surgeons are already experiencing great satisfaction from implementing this form of conservative care when missed by the referring source that turned out to be so successful in bringing about recovery. Surgeons who already incorporate MDT in their surgical selection process are not only pleased about what it has added, but find that patients leaving their care to return to their community and referring doctor spread the word about the rapid recovery and successful care they received based on the recommendation of their surgeon.

Alternatively, for those surgical candidates who turn out to be non-centralizers with no directional preference when examined by a Credentialed or Diplomaed MDT clinician, surgeons can be assured that conservative care is one important step closer to truly being exhausted and also reinforced by the outstanding surgical outcomes for non-centralizers reported in at least two studies.[56, 80]

Some spine surgeons have also appreciated the value of promoting the use of MDT to their referring physicians to be implemented prior to referral in hopes of avoiding unnecessary referrals to the surgeon that consume spots on the surgeon's office schedule that could be filled by more legitimate, post-MDT, surgical candidates. This in turn decreases the surgeon's new patient wait times and decreases the number of patient visits required to find a surgical case.

In consideration of surgeons' and hospitals' incomes, a very important and sensitive topic, this seems to be quite similar to the dental profession championing the means of preventing dental caries (tooth decay) through effective prophylaxis. Caring for dental cavities was once dentistry's bread-and-butter. There were widespread concerns within the profession that they might even put themselves out of business. Yet today, they continue to thrive economically, performing many other dental procedures while continuing to promote the importance of prophylaxis for their patients' dental health. I have no doubt that there will remain plenty of spinal surgery still to do, but its indications and patient-selection process will become much more precise, improving outcomes while avoiding unnecessary surgeries.

Payers/Employers: Payers, especially large self-insured employers, have a huge LBP overhead, but they also often have some ability to influence the type of care their employees with LBP pursue. Consequently, with so much of their cost being unnecessary, these employers have great incentive to find ways to "help MDT happen" as early in the care of their employees and dependants as possible. Doing so also provides them with objective, evidence-based assessment information that can guide their decision-making about what interventions will be productive and which ones will not, while helping most become independent of the need for long term or repetitive care.

From a payer and societal economic perspective, this would appear to be a no-brainer: finding a way to empower individuals with LBP to take control of, and even eliminate, their own pain using a low-tech outpatient intervention emphasizing education and self-care.

In the absence of actual cost-saving data, let's consider these numbers. If 70% of acute LBP patients have a directional preference and can abolish their own pain, along with up to 50% of those currently recommended for disc surgery,[50, 80, 82] and if many can also learn how to prevent or reduce the number of their recurrences,[81] it is not outlandish to estimate that the broad utilization of this MDT paradigm as the entry point for low back care could generate a 50% savings in LBP costs. That has yet to be tested and quantified of course, and such widespread utilization is completely unrealistic for many reasons, but from a societal perspective, with an estimated annual LBP overhead in the U.S. of $90B, savings that fall far short of 50% would still be extraordinary.

Researchers: The very thing that so many research experts have been calling essential over the past eight years is happening. The validation of LBP subgroups provides a whole new foundation and direction for research over the next ten years simply by studying the directional preference/centralizing subgroup whose recovery is so common and predictable using end-range directional loading strategies. How to understand and manage the other, relatively small, yet still important, subgroups in which a directional preference is not found, is yet another goldmine. While the LBP black box will likely always exist, it is shrinking as each pain response subgroup is validated and removed from it.

A re-read of Chapter 11 will provide a further review of many forms of clinical research that are ready to be undertaken.

The Disease Management Industry: I mentioned this combination of patient education and self-care accountability in Chapter 10. The economic value of identifying and implementing validated self-care is immense and is being appreciated more and more within the business world. Alvin Toffler, author of *Revolutionary Wealth*[24,][138] states: "Everyone has gotten excited about outsourcing to India or China. But nobody has paid attention to the outsourcing from the company to the customer. We do our own banking using ATM machines, track our FedEx packages on the Internet, and act as our own online travel agents. We're told that these changes benefit us. And some do. But the transfer of labor from paid employees to unpaid consumers allows companies to significantly reduce their work forces." When was the last time someone filled your car's gas tank for you or you talked to a bank teller? Toffler refers to our future economy as one where almost everyone participates. Should health care be any different?

This is just what disease management companies are attempting to do within health care: transferring responsibility for effective proactive self-care to patients, thereby reducing the costs of care, especially the occurrence of later complications, and preventing the development of more advanced disease using more interactive educational technologies.

I spoke in Chapter 10 about a web-based interactive educational program we've developed which brings LBP patients important baseline understanding of how to eliminate their own back problems as well as expedite, when necessary, their access to the specialized care of MDT-trained and other specialists. It enables the significant time required for patient education in individualized self-care to be transferred to the patient without tying up a professional's time. Expediting knowledge transfer in this way enables disease management companies, with its telephonic workforce, to serve far greater volumes of LBP sufferers using evidence-based content.

Prior to this book, based on their unfamiliarity with the MDT assessment, self-care methods, and its abundant supportive evidence, most disease management companies and LBP economists have been constrained in their program development by the feeble, one-size-fits-all recommendations of most guidelines. Alternatively, a LBP disease management program designed around patient empowerment through individualized self-care offers very attractive, cost-effective alternatives.

I predict MDT-based self-care education will emerge as an economic boon for disease management companies and their large employer customers. The use of the MDT paradigm can leverage this ability to reliably assess and classify patients along with interactive web-based infrastructure and educational models to greatly reduce program operating costs and improve clinical outcomes, while substantially decreasing customers' (i.e. employers') costs of low back care.

The compelling goal for all LBP stakeholders should be to help as many patients as possible to become pain-free and independent of the health care system. The fact that this can be done by determining and then showing people how they can eliminate their own pain is the key to success. Substantial cost-reduction follows by eliminating the need for further diagnostic and therapeutic interventions and the associated disability.

Consequently, every LBP sufferer, or at least those not responding after some designated period of time, deserves the opportunity to have this inexpensive, highly informative, MDT assessment. How can we justify withholding the opportunity for patients to learn how to reduce or eliminate their own pain and disability? On one hand, we routinely pay for expensive, high-tech diagnostic and therapeutic innovations that are often short on evidence of effectiveness, meanwhile failing to encourage the use of this low-tech, low-cost intervention capable of obviating the need for so many expensive LBP interventions.

Who can help it happen?

Without exception, all LBP stakeholders can play a role in hastening the spread of MDT innovation.

Clinicians are often perceived to be slow to change their practice patterns, although either a threat of loss or a chance of enhancement to their livelihood understandably grabs their attention, motivating them to make practice changes much more readily. Changes in reimbursement or changes in patient demands and their provider selection (i.e., voting with their feet) all greatly affect clinicians' behavior.

Meanwhile, most LBP clinicians remain either unfamiliar with, or simply misunderstand, MDT. And there is certainly no financial incentive for them to become interested. Frankly, most family physicians are just too busy and have too much else to do to try to learn or even keep up with one more thing.

However, once patients and payers understand that such successful self-care is available at such low cost, further incentives will motivate some clinicians to seek education and to alter their practice patterns.

Researchers must also reconsider their work, not that they should have an agenda to help implement MDT but, consistent with their role in designing and carrying out credible trials with valid conclusions, they need to begin to incorporate the A–D–T–O model into their clinical research designs even as they re-consider the existing literature that includes reliability, predictive cohort studies, and both black box and the recent subgroup-specific RCTs. Given the widespread consensus that identifying and validating LBP subgroups is a high priority, moving to the A–D–T–O research model would seem to be a priority.

Employers and health plans stand to benefit substantially from finding ways to stimulate the availability, accessibility and use of the MDT assessment and treatment. In an ideal world, it should be provided to every LBP sufferer early in their care.

How to help it happen

Based on the evidence we've reviewed throughout this book, the benefit of having more LBP patients undergoing the MDT assessment earlier in their care seems evident in order to classify them and direct their subsequent care.

Let's explore five important areas intended to "help MDT happen":

1. better compensation for appropriately trained clinicians
2. investing in the education of LBP clinicians
3. helping more patients access MDT assessment and self-care as indicated
4. re-structuring LBP research to focus much more on subgroup identification and understanding
5. replacing "the diagnostic triage" in clinical guidelines, with its acknowledged lack of evidence, with a recognition of the evidence supporting pain response classification, including centralization and directional preference, as reliable, highly predictive of outcomes, and with efficacy evidence in multiple RCTs.

1. Better compensation for MDT-trained clinicians

PERSONAL DISCLOSURE: *While I am personally qualified at the Diploma level of MDT, I am neither practicing medicine nor do I have any financial relationship with any clinics who would financially benefit from what I am about to propose.*

A significant obstacle to the greater availability of the MDT assessment is the limited number of fully trained clinicians in the medical, physical therapy, osteopathic and chiropractic disciplines. This obstacle is in large part tied to the lack of any financial incentive to undertake the extensive time and financial requirements to become fully trained and credentialed. Payers currently spend tens of thousands of dollars for new innovative surgical procedures with limited evidence of efficacy without realizing the strong evidence that, for a few hundred dollars for an MDT assessment, many LBP patients, including surgical candidates, can recover quite simply, even rapidly.

Unfortunately, reimbursement is the same for an MDT assessment as it is for an examination that only calls for having a patient bend forward and backward once and then conducting a simple lower extremity neurological exam. The latter takes only one or two minutes but, more importantly, provides such limited information that it often is the first step in mismanagement of their low back condition. At the risk of redundancy, recall once again the Quebec Task Force's conclusion: "There is so much variability in making a diagnosis that this initial step routinely introduces inaccuracies which are then further confounded with each succeeding step in care." The resulting diagnosis "is the fundamental source of error."[132] How many patients are directed to treatment interventions and expensive tests based on such a brief and uninformative physical evaluation?

Alternatively, the MDT assessment routinely requires 15–30 minutes depending on the complexity of each patient, followed by the essential need to explain the relevance of the pain response findings, then teach and justify the patient's self-treatment exercises and posture strategies (another 10–20 minutes). Unfortunately, there is no billing code that in any way properly reflects this much assessment time or this level of expertise.

To date, only physical therapists have committed to the MDT paradigm in any large numbers, although more and more members of the chiropractic profession are seeking training. There is unfortunately only a very small number of MDs who have taken MDT courses and only a handful of us who have reached the Credentialed or Diploma level. I believe this training should be an essential part of any clinician who is seeing and managing LBP patients with any regularity, regardless of health care discipline.

In order to attract more clinicians in all disciplines to this form of care, practitioners must see realistic incentives to justify and motivate their investment of time and money to pursue the proper coursework and then attain the Credentialed or Diploma level of MDT proficiency (see Chapter 13).

So what specific incentives could be provided to motivate clinicians to seek this training?

A. Higher reimbursement for an MDT assessment conducted by a Credentialed or Diplomate in MDT. This would likely require the creation and use of a unique billing code for the MDT *assessment*. This is a complex undertaking requiring powerful organizations to sponsor new codes, yet payers need to be aware of the benefits of doing so. On the treatment side, MDT's focus on exercise prescriptions and education is more easily represented by existing procedure (CPT) codes in the U.S. and therefore new treatment codes are not as important or necessary.

B. Another payment model that would benefit both payers and MDT clinicians is some form of "pay-for-performance" program. Generally, MDT practitioners can achieve their good and excellent outcomes in fewer visits (most average 5–6 visits) than most other treatment paradigms. Such a program would require establishing criteria to define successful outcomes as well as negotiating the number of visits.

2. Invest in MDT education

A. Spread the word. I believe the information provided in this book is vital to reforming how we understand, research and care for LBP. It is my hope that this book will be widely read as an educational tool by employer health personnel, health plans, clinicians, and researchers.

B. Subsidize the cost of MDT education for clinicians. It is no doubt premature to think about making MDT training and credentialing compulsory in order to manage LBP patients. However, there is a case to be made for payers, particularly employers, to encourage, even subsidize, the cost of MDT education and completion of the credentialing examination for interested medical doctors, osteopaths, physical therapists and chiropractors in their communities. Providing scholarships would not only attract clinicians to this educational process and help make this important assessment more accessible, but it would also help shrink the pool of clinicians currently providing unreliable and unvalidated assessment exams. Both of these elements would contribute to improving outcomes and lowering the cost of low back care. This very strategy of providing scholarships has been proposed to employers by Thomas Friedman in his national bestseller *The World Is Flat* in an effort to stimulate U.S. college education in the sciences in order to remain competitive in our rapidly changing global economy.[61]

3. Help more patients access MDT assessment

Back in Chapter 10, we discussed three specific advantageous times to steer LBP patients toward an MDT assessment, concluding that the-earlier-the-better was the most cost-effective thing to do.

A. Pre-surgery MDT assessment. You'll recall the three studies that report that 32–50% of disc surgery candidates are actually centralizers.[50, 80, 82] Given the high rates of recoveries for this large subgroup, even at an apparently recalcitrant stage of disc disorder, the cost savings implications of avoiding this many surgeries are huge. Spending for lumbar spinal fusions has increased more than 500% over the past decade and now represents 40% of all low back care spending[154].

Indeed, there are no doubt many patients undergoing disc surgery unnecessarily with excellent and fairly rapid outcomes anticipated if their non-surgical treatment was determined by the directional preference found during their MDT assessment.[56, 65, 72, 88, 90, 129, 136, 157, 158] Note also that these rapid recoveries[90] contrast greatly with the slow non-surgical improvements that can take a year or more currently described to patients as their most attractive alternative to surgery as part of shared-decision-making discussions. What a pity that pre-surgical patients who have the good fortune to be provided with cutting edge shared-decision-making video presentations still never hear anything about the possibility that they may still have a rapidly reversible problem that first may just need detecting in order to discover how they can bring about their own recovery.

In an effort to avoid these unnecessary disc surgeries, most spine surgeons would seem willing, if not eager, to provide his or her patients with an MDT evaluation. The problem is that most surgeons remain unfamiliar with centralization, directional preference, the strength of the supportive evidence, and the need for well-trained examiners.

Alternatively, many payers, armed with this information, may decide to exercise the option of requiring such an assessment prior to authorizing any lumbar disc surgery. Not only will they potentially save the cost of the surgery, but the costs of complications, failed or only partially successful surgery, the 10–15% chance of a re-operation, and costs of any persisting disability. We must also appreciate that identifying a centralizer, who then goes on to a good outcome, saves the money that would have been spent on subsequent non-operative care if they had chosen to pass up surgery.

B. Chronic, non-surgical patients. Even chronic LBP patients who are not considered surgical candidates may be undetected centralizers. One study assessed patients at the outset of their chronic LBP rehabilitation program reporting that 43% were centralizers.[88] So, if not previously assessed, there is excellent reason to provide all chronic LBP patients the opportunity to undergo an MDT assessment with a well-trained clinician.

I cannot overemphasize this point about the value of a well-trained clinician. So many lesser trained practitioners to whom your chronic patient may have previously been referred claim to know and use McKenzie methods but I cannot tell you how many times patients with persisting LBP who had previously been referred for McKenzie care and evaluated by a non-credentialed practitioner, then centralized and recovered nicely once I referred them to a Credentialed or Diplomaed MDT clinician.

Consequently, if a chronic rehabilitation program does not have a Credentialed MDT clinician on staff to provide this assessment, the payer would be wise to arrange for such an evaluation prior to commencing such a rehab program. This same prospective cohort study concluded that the management of centralizers in their chronic rehab program was very different from non-centralizing patients because centralizers had the distinct advantage of being able to control and even abolish their pain, enabling them to return to work sooner than the non-centralziers.[88]

C. Acute and subacute patients. We must also keep in mind that the prevalence of centralization and directional preference is considerably higher in acute and subacute LBP than in chronic, yet so many remain undetected and symptomatic as a result of never being assessed to discover their directional preference. With 70–80% of acute care-seekers being centralizers, members of this large group have no need for any diagnostic studies, prolonged non-operative care, any invasive treatments, and should have little if any disability.

While it is unrealistic at this time for payers to steer all acute LBP care seekers to MDT clinicians for assessment, it may be appropriate to think about how much unsuccessful treatment time should be allowed to elapse before such an assessment is considered, encouraged, or even required. The published data make a strong case of requiring the MDT assessment before authorizing any big ticket items, such as advanced imaging, spinal injections or discography, none of which centralizers typically need. Further, because so many acute and subacute patients are taking various medications to help them control their pain, some of them addicting, both the expense and the risk of these side-effects justify exploring MDT's low-tech means of gaining control of, and even eliminating, the pain and the underlying problem using reliably identified self-treatment interventions.

4. Re-structure LBP research to focus much more

on subgroup identification and understanding

Of course, inherent in all this is the need to pursue and encourage much more productive research: to specifically explore the goldmine related to validated subgroups.

We could start with centralizers and non-centralizers, justified by the substantial clinical validation of these subgroups (see Chapter 8). LBP clinical research also needs to shift to the A–D–T–O model and stop wasting limited research funds on black box RCTs focused on non-specific LBP. We should also be encouraging clinicians of all disciplines to first demonstrate their abilities, or lack thereof, to produce inter-examiner reliability with their assessment methods.

Another very exciting branch of this goldmine is the basic science directed at exploring the underlying mechanisms of centralization, non-centralization, and directional preferences. Are these pain responses tied to a symptom-generating disc or are there other anatomic sources and mechanisms?

Payers can also participate in research, even in-house research. Many employers and health plans already have the means of validating the savings of this paradigm for their own employees or subscribers. By determining which of their LBP providers are McKenzie-trained (see Chapter 13) and which are not enables a query of their database to determine the number of LBP clinic or office visits with each type of clinician. This usually reveals a significant difference with Credentialed McKenzie practitioners usually averaging just 5–6 visits per patient while non-McKenzie care typically takes two or three times as many visits, sometimes even more. Comparing MDT outcomes with others' outcomes, while important, is not as easy.

Payers can also play an important role in supporting quality low back research by helping to fund it, probably done most easily through appropriate research foundations. One such recently formed foundation already has an appreciation for the importance of the A–D–T–O research model. The International Mechanical Diagnosis and Therapy Research Foundation is completely independent from the McKenzie Institute and its mission statement is "To fund original research world-wide that contributes to the body of evidence related to the usefulness and limitations of Mechanical Diagnosis and Therapy."

5. Replace "the diagnostic triage"

Implausibly, LBP clinical guidelines continue to advocate the diagnostic triage as a means of LBP classification, despite it having no supportive evidence,[143] while continuing to ignore the considerable evidence supporting the reliability and validity for both the MDT and Delitto classification systems.

Making it happen?

A word about "making it happen." While not so common, this is perhaps most often observed as an administrative effort. I do see a time, perhaps sooner rather than later, where LBP clinicians may be required by payers to provide this form of assessment by referral if not personally. Such a requirement would be justified by the potential for avoiding a situation where a centralizer with a good prognosis with proper treatment would remain unrecognized or receive ineffective or even counterproductive treatment.[90]

Chapter 16

Where Have We Been and Where Are You Going?

*Honest criticism is hard to take, particularly from
a relative, a friend, an acquaintance, or a stranger.*
                                        —*Benjamin Franklin.*

We're nearing the completion of our journey together. It's been an interesting, enjoyable and certainly challenging time for me to commit this information and my thoughts gathered over twenty-five years into a (I hope) coherent text. I sincerely hope that the journey has been interesting and worthwhile for you, perhaps even challenging.

We started by discussing the tension between low back researchers and clinicians over clinical guidelines, all rooted in our inability to make a diagnosis in the majority of LBP cases. That single deficiency has led us through decades of research that has viewed LBP as though most suffer from the same type of non-specific problem. Meanwhile, most clinicians persist in their attempts to somehow classify their LBP patients using questionably reliable, or even unreliable and therefore invalid, distinctions that too often serve the clinician as much as the patient in justifying the use of favored treatments.

David Eddy wrote: "The plain fact is that many decisions made by physicians appear to be arbitrary—highly variable, with no obvious explanation. The very disturbing implication is that this arbitrariness represents, for at least some patients, suboptimal or even harmful care."[57] We've certainly seen data showing that suboptimal, harmful care can occur, even with so-called "evidence-based care."

Someone else has said: "Yesterday's wisdom is today's folly." The information I've brought to you hopefully represents some of today's wisdom and even some of its folly, fulfilling many experts' views that identifying and establishing LBP subgroups should be our top priority in advancing our understanding of LBP and its management. That fulfillment is based on the scientific evidence establishing both the inter-examiner reliability of the MDT assessment and the ability of its findings to identify subgroup-specific treatments that substantially improve outcomes for most, while also predicting poor outcomes and the need for more extensive care for a much smaller LBP subgroup. The centralization/directional preference subgroup comprises a very large portion of acute LBP and a smaller, but still very important, portion of chronic LBP. The recent emergence of four favorable RCTs further validates this form of assessment, patient classification, and subgroup-specific treatment.

I am unable to fully explain why the MDT paradigm has so consistently been either misrepresented or just plain overlooked by international experts and clinical guideline panelists for so long. But I suspect it is tied to a mix of divergent, even misdirected, research agendas with an excessive focus on RCTs, particularly black box RCTs, further mixed with a commonplace dose of large egos, professional jealousies, and economic considerations, any of which can blur objectivity in the best of us. However, in some cases, it seems to also be tied to closed minds unwilling to "hear" presentations made or read correspondence written that clearly points out that MDT is not just extension exercises but an assessment that determines a patient-specific treatment.

Meanwhile, there are so many motivated, skilled researchers around the world who can and, no doubt, will contribute greatly to our LBP understanding if they are willing to have a more open mind about the things I have presented in this book. I predict it will be a great and grand journey for those who do shift their focus to first understanding and then expanding on the existing research targeting MDT care.

Although there is an enormous amount of exciting research ahead of us, there is already a broad foundation of evidence to justify what, for many, is a whole new paradigm of low back care. It was a call for a new paradigm after all that was listed back in 1998 as one of the top ten LBP research priorities.[14] There is good and still increasing evidence that pain response classifications, especially centralization, provide the means for identifying validated subgroups.[32]

Given this extensive published evidence validating centralization and directional preference, clinicians, researchers, systematic reviewers and guideline panelists alike who continue to view MDT as only an exercise treatment will now, more than ever, continue to expose their lack of understanding of this approach, which is not a responsible position for acclaimed experts.

To be sure, MDT is not a panacea for LBP. It is therefore a mistake to interpret MDT clinicians' enthusiasm for this clinical approach to be an indication that they believe they can fix everyone. It is just the opposite in fact. One of the basic explanations for MDT clinicians' enthusiasm is their ability and confidence in determining quite early just who they *cannot* treat with this approach. To not understand this about MDT clinicians again exposes one's incomplete understanding of this paradigm.

Pursuing that same line of thought, in order to ensure and sustain credibility in today's spine care marketplace, clinicians who advocate specific LBP treatments are obliged to accurately define their clinical limitations and indications for referral of their patients for other care rather than just prolonging or indiscriminately changing their own treatments in hopes of finding something that might work.

Consequently, for these same clinicians who advocate non-MDT LBP paradigms, there is value in re-examining any literature directed at their own LBP assessments and classification methods for reliability and validity, consistent with the first two links of the A–D–T–O model. We earlier cited Maier's Law: if facts conflict with a theory, either the theory must be changed, or the facts. How many clinicians using either unreliable or untested assessments are willing to revise their LBP management methods to align with the extensive evidence that most LBP patients have a directional preference enabling subgroup classification and specific treatment? Or do they discard this evidence in order to remain loyal to their unreliable or untested assessment process, as well as their unproven but favorite pain-generating theories, disease models, and dogma inherent with the traditions of the discipline?

Employers and health plans meanwhile genuinely seek to improve their employees' and members' low back care as a means of reducing their high overhead. They know that quality care is cost-effective care. But they have understandably sought direction from clinical guideline recommendations about what form of low back care to purchase. But we have seen the large differences between guideline-based and evidence-based care, with considerable evidence outside the guidelines that provides valuable assistance in cutting costs while also improving their employees' and members' outcomes. It is uncertain just when guidelines will catch up to this evidence.

Over the years, many LBP experts have questioned the balance, or lack thereof, with which I have weighed the MDT evidence. I strive to be objective, like everyone else does, and I find that no one is without some bias, whether intentional or not, including researchers who claim to be fully evidence-based.

That question about me then begs an examination of the balance, or lack thereof, of those concerned about me. The irony is that many of these experts persist in their mistaken view of MDT as just extension exercises despite its 25 years of educational availability and all its supportive evidence. These same individuals are also part of the guideline consensus that recommends the "diagnostic triage" for classifying acute LBP, despite its acknowledged lack of evidence, yet continue to avoid any recognition of the many supportive reliability, classification, and outcome predictive studies. They further claim that LBP has a highly favorable LBP natural history, failing any mention of data that challenges this view. Finally, they routinely acknowledge, dare I say promote, the role of psychosocial yellow flags as obstacles to recovery and predictors of poor outcomes, completely disregarding the many studies documenting the ability of baseline pain response findings (centralization, directional preference, or their absence) to predict either strongly favorable or poor outcomes.

By writing this book, I have been able to share the evidence as well as expand on it with my views of the importance and many positive consequences of being able to reliably identify and validate LBP subgroups. I am also aware that the enthusiasm I held for MDT 25 years ago has not dissipated. The big difference is that today my views and enthusiasm have been vindicated by the comprehensive A–D–T–O evidence for MDT care. My views are no longer based on my and others' anecdotal experiences. This evidence is clear and growing, enabling us to now solve large portions of the non-specific-LBP puzzle while also decreasing the high costs of low back care. Enthusiasm backed by scientific evidence does not constitute bias. Indeed, such evidence should generate enthusiasm in anyone truly seeking cost-effective LBP solutions. Observing patients' reactions to their pain centralizing and abolishing during the performance of a repetitive end-range exercise is so often an eye- and mind-opener.

Consequently, I hope this book will nudge, perhaps even drive, open-minded solution-seekers, whether they are patients, clinicians, researchers, or payers, toward incorporating this MDT paradigm into their clinical or research approach to LBP. It is my expectation that the wider utilization of MDT by properly trained clinicians will produce the same satisfying clinical results we've been discussing throughout this book, creating even more satisfaction and enthusiasm over the ability to genuinely and positively affect the course and cost of LBP.

In closing, consider these five "help it happen" strategies:

1. Help disseminate this important information regarding MDT low back care and the A–D–T–O research model I've presented in this book.
2. Encourage, sponsor, and even require MDT education in order to provide this care early and conveniently for all your LBP employees, members and patients.
3. Help fund, and even participate in, LBP research that follows the A–D–T–O research model or that further explores the validity and pain-generating mechanisms of various subgroups, especially the very large subgroup whose pain centralizes with a directional preference who can rapidly recover.
4. Encourage, even require, the MDT assessment prior to any diagnostic or treatment referrals tied to any significant expense.
5. Find ways to financially reward credentialed MDT clinicians for their lengthy and extensive training that can bring this scientifically validated clinical care to more LBP sufferers, as well as motivating other clinicians to seek this same training.

There now remains just one more important question: what will you personally do with all this information as you proceed with your efforts to provide more LBP relief and cost savings within your own sphere of influence?

Never doubt that a small group of thoughtful, committed citizens
can change the world. Indeed, it's the only thing that ever has.
                                                    —*Margaret Mead*

Appendix: Pain Response Clinical Studies

The following tables summarize various pain response clinical studies categorized by their study design and topic. These categories are: reliability studies, cohort, prevalence and outcome prediction studies, randomized clinical trials (some focusing on "directional" treatment interventions and others on efficacy of care based on pain response assessment), and studies attempting to correlate pain response patterns with disc pathology.

Reliability studies focused on pain response testing and patient classification

Study	Participants	Design/Methods	Results	Conclusions
Spratt K, Lehmann T, Weinstein J, Sayre H **A new approach to the low back physical examination: behavioral assessment of mechanical signs** Spine 15:96-102, 1990	42 pts with LBP were assigned to one of three rater pairs trained in the examination methods.	A test-retest paradigm of 17 organic tests and 4 non-organic tests. Tests included single and repeated standing and recumbent trunk flexion & extension, seated and supine SLR, back tenderness, femoral nerve stretch and instability test.	Pts reports of pain location were quite stable across examinations but reports of pain aggravation were generally less consistent across time than were rater observed pain behaviors. The reliability for the organic and non-organic pain behavior composites were 0.78 and 0.82 respectively.	The physical exam produces useful examiner-based outcome measures to supplement or complement traditional patient self-report measures of outcome.
Kilby J, Stigant M, Roberts **The reliability of back pain assessment by physiotherapists, using a "McKenzie algorithm"** Physiotherapy, 1990 76:579-83.	41 patients with LBP	Pts examined by two therapists according to an algorithm of McK assessment.	The algorithm was reliable in examination of pain behavior and pain response with repeated movement, but unreliable in the detection of end-range pain, presence of kyphotic or flat lumbar spine and relevant lateral shift.	The algorithm's primary use is as a research tool for examination of inter-therapist agreement.

Study	Participants	Design/Methods	Results	Conclusions
Riddle D, Rothstein J Intertester reliability of McKenzie's classification of the syndrome types present in patients with low back pain. Spine 18:1333-44, 1993	363 pts. with LBP were examined by randomly paired PTs in 8 clinics. 33 of 49 PTs had no formal McKenzie training.	*Examiners with little/no McK training* given summary of McK evaluation and criteria used to classify patients. Pts examined separately by two randomly assigned PTs. Kappa coefficient values determined.	Percent agreement was 39% and K = 0.26. For PTs with some post-graduate training in the McK system, K = 0.15 and the percentage agreement = 27%.	Poor inter-tester reliability reported using examiners with little training.
Sufka A, Hauger B, Trenary M, et al. **Centralization of low back pain and perceived functional outcome.** Journal of Orthopedics and Sports Physical Therapy, 1998. 27(3): 205-12.	36 LBP patients w/ or w/o leg pain. Pain duration: QTFI: 6, QTF2: 15, QTF3: 15 Pain location: QTFI: 15 (back pain only), QTF2: 7, QTF3: 14 (below knee)	All patients evaluated with McKenzie methods. Treatment based on McK assessment findings. Outcomes: Oswestry, Spinal Function Sort at baseline and 14-day FU.	94% agreement/inter-rater reliability w/ centralization in pilot group. Complete centralization occurred in 69% over 14 days (mean=4.3): acute=83%, subacute=73% & chronic= 60% / QTFI=80%, QTF2-73%, QTF3 =43%. Fewer chronics and fewer w/ pain below the knee completely centralized.	LBP sufferers show greater improvement (functional outcomes) when there is evidence of "complete" centralization within 14 days than when there is not. Time of complete centralization was no longer for chronics or those with pain below the knee.
Wilson L, Hall H, McIntosh G, Melles T Intertester reliability of a low back pain classification system Spine 24:248-54, 1999	204 pts. with LBP referred to 10 clinics	Paired PTs performed separate exams consisting of movement testing and pain response monitoring and chose one of five pain patterns. % agreement and Kappa values determined.	Agreement in classification was 78.9% with Kappa = 0.61.	Physiotherapists trained in a classification system based on monitoring of pain patterns during movement testing of pts with LBP demonstrated high inter-tester reliability.
Werneke M, Hart D, Cook D. **A descriptive study of the centralization phenomenon: a prospective analysis.** Spine, 1999. 24: 676-83.	289 consecutive patients with acute neck or LBP with or without referred spinal symptoms referred to PT.	Subjects assessed & categorized into 3 pain pattern groups using McK assessment. Pain location & intensity, functional status, # treatment visits compared between the 3 groups.	Inter-tester reliability between judges: excellent for distal pain location and classification. Cent'zers (partial & full)-77%, non-cent'zers- 23%. Cent'zers had significantly fewer visits (p<0.001), less pain intensity and better function (p<0.001) than other groups	Categorization by change in pain location to mechanical assessment allowed identification of patients with improved outcomes and facilitated treatment planning for those in need of more extensive evaluations

Study	Participants	Design/Methods	Results	Conclusions
Razmjou H, Kramer J, Yamada, R **Intertester reliability of the McKenzie evaluation in assessing patients with mechanical low back pain** J, Ortho & Sports Phys Ther 30:368-89, 2000	45 pts. presenting to physical therapy with acute, subacute or chronic LBP.	Each pt. was examined simultaneously by two PTs, both trained in the McK evaluation system. One PT was the assessor, the other an observer. Examiners classified each pt. by syndrome, sub-syndrome, presence and relevance of lateral shift, relevance of lateral component, and sagittal deformity.	Agreement for syndrome selection was Kappa = 0.70; for derangement sub-syndromes K = 0.96; for presence of lateral shift K = 0.52, relevance of lateral shift K = 0.85, relevance of lateral component K = 0.95, and deformity in sagittal plane was K = 1.00. For the 17 pts. under 55 yr old, agreement on syndrome categories was K = 1.00.	This form of low back evaluation using patterns of pain response to repeated end-range test movements was highly reliable when performed by two well-trained physical therapists.
Fritz J, Delitto A, Vignovic M, Busse R **Interrater reliability of judgements of the central'n phenomenon and status change during movement testing in patients with low back pain** Archives of Physical Med & Rehab 81:57-61, 2000	Pts. receiving phys. ther. for low back pain were videotaped. 40 licensed phys therapists and 40 P.T. students served as subjects in viewing videotapes of pt. examinations.	A videotape study of judgments of the 80 clinician viewers of the results of single, repeated, & sustained movement testing of pts. with LBP regarding whether pts. pain centralized, peripheral-ized, or remained status quo. Percentage agreement and Kappa coefficient values were determined.	Inter-rater reliability was excellent for the total sample of examiners (K = 0.793), for licensed PTs (K = .823), and for students (K = .763).	Judgments of status change are reliable when operational definitions are provided. Clinical experience did not substantially improve reliability with the use of precise operational definitions.
Kilpikoski S, Airaksinen O, Kankaanpää M, Leminen P, Videman T, Alen FM **Interexaminer reliability in low back pain assessment using the McKenzie method.** Spine, 2002. 27: E207-14	39 volunteers with low back pain, mean age 40 years (range, 24–55 years)	Test-retest design. LBP pts. blindly assessed by two PTs well-trained in McK methods. % agreement and Kappa coefficient calculated.	Agreement in identifying the central-ization phenomenon and directional preference was 95% (kappa = 0.7; P < 0.002) and 90% (K = 0.9; P < 0.000), respectively, and in classifying patients into McKenzie main syndromes and into specific subgroups was 95% (K = 0.6; P < 0.000) and 74% (K = 0.7; P < 0.000), respectively.	Inter-examiner reliability of McK lumbar tests and classifying patients into syndromes were high and statistically significant when the examiners had been trained in the McK method.

Study	Participants	Design/Methods	Results	Conclusions
Clare H, Adams R, Maher C **Reliability of McKenzie classification of patients with cervical and lumbar pain.** J. Manip & Physiolog'l Therap'cs, 2005. 28:122-7.	25 pts with lumbar and 25 with cervical pain	Pts were assessed simultaneously by 2 PTs (14 in total) trained in the McKenzie method. Agreement was expressed using the multi-rater Kappa coefficient and percent agreement for classification into (i) syndromes and (ii) sub-syndromes.	For syndrome classification: K = 0.84 with 96% agreement for the total patient pool, K = 1.0 with 100% agreement for lumbar and K = 0.63 with 92% agreement for cervical patients. For sub-syndrome classification: K = 0.87 with 90% agreement for the total patient pool, K = 0.89 with 92% agreement for lumbar patients, and K = 0.64 with 88% agreement for the cervical patients.	The McKenzie assessment performed by clinicians trained in the McKenzie method may allow for reliable classification of patients with lumbar and cervical pain.
Fritz J, Brennan G, Shannon N, Clifford S, Hunter S, Thackeray A **An examination of the reliability of a classification algorithm for subgrouping patients with low back pain.** Spine, 2006. 31:77-82.	60 LBP pts of less than 90 days duration participated whose pain remained stable between examinations: mean age 37.7, 44% female	Pts examined on separate days by different examiners with findings used to classify patients using the decision-making algorithm *by clinicians with varying amounts of experience.* Inter-rater reliability of individual exam items for classification examined using Kappa coefficients and intra-class correlation coefficients.	Reliability of range of motion, centralization/ peripheralization judgments with flexion and extension, and the instability test were moderate to excellent. Reliability of centralization/ peripheralization judgments with repeated or sustained extension or aberrant movement judgments was fair to poor. Overall agreement on classification decisions was 76% (kappa = 0.60, 95% confidence interval 0.56, 0.64), with no significant differences based on level of experience.	Reliability of the classification algorithm was good. Further research is needed to identify sources of disagreements and improve reproducibility.

Cohort, Prevalence, and Outcome Prediction Studies

Study	Participants	Design/Methods	Results	Conclusions
Kopp J, Alexander A, Turocy R, Levrini M, Lichtman D **The use of lumbar extension in the evaluation and treatment of patients with acute herniated nucleus pulposus, a preliminary report** Clinical Orthopedics, 1986. 202:211-8.	67 pts. with LBP radiating to the calf or foot with at least one significant sign of nerve root irritation and at least 6 wks of failed non-operative therapy.	All pts. underwent an initial trial of extension exercises. Those who had no symptom worsening were prescribed an extension exercise program for several days while still hospitalized.	34 (52%) experienced no symptom worsening during extension tests. All 34 performed extension exercise program. 100% regained their full lumbar extension range and eliminated symptoms within 2-5 days. The other 32 underwent laminectomy and discectomy. Pre-operatively, there was no difference between the groups with regard to age, gender, pain below the knee, or any of the neurological signs or SLR. 56% of the surgical patients had a free fragment, 19% had a swollen of displaced nerve root, and 19% had a bulging disc.	"Some of these patients responded so dramatically to extension therapy that the use of extension exercises as a therapeutic modality is recommended."
Donelson R, Silva G, Murphy K. **The centralization phenomenon: its usefulness in evaluating and treating referred pain** Spine, 1990. 15(3): 211-13	87 patients with LBP and radiating leg pain presenting to a general orthopedic practice. Pain duration: 53 acutes (0-4 wks), 15 subacutes (4-12 wks), 19 chronics (12+ wks.)	Independent retrospective chart review. Patients all assessed and/or treated with McKenzie form of care. Presence or absence of centralization on initial assessment correlated with treatment outcomes. Outcomes at time of discharge: pain relief, return to activity/work, patient satisfaction.	Centralization occurred in 87% (89/87/84% of acutes, subacutes, chronics). 98/77/81% of centralizers, 17/50/33% of non-centralizers had good or excellent outcomes. Only 4 surgical disc patients: all were non-centralizers and all did well with surgery.	Centralization occurred commonly and its presence or absence was a strong predictor of treatment outcome and the presence or absence of surgical disc pathology.
Long A **The centralization phenomenon: its usefulness as a predictor of outcome in conservative treatment of chronic low back pain.** Spine, 1995. 20(23): 2513-21.	223 chronic LBP patients presenting to interdisciplinary rehab facility, all receiving compensation.	All assessed with McKenzie methods with each patient classified as a centralizer or non-centralizer. Treatment 5 days/wk for 11 wks of work hardening, work simulation, exercise, P.T., psychological support. Outcomes: Pain intensity, lifting capacity, Oswestry, RTW status at 9 mon and 2 yrs.	Centralization occurred in 47% of patients. Centralizers: greater decrease in pain intensity (p=0.05) and higher RTW rate (p=0.034). No difference in Oswestry scores and lift capacity.	Centralizers had better outcomes with treatment than non-centralizers. Identifying centralizat'n can be used to identify subgroups with different prognoses or treatment requirements.

Study	Participants	Design/Methods	Results	Conclusions
Karas R, McIntosh G, Hall H, et al. **The relationship between non-organic signs and centralization of symptoms in the prediction of return to work for patients with low back pain.** Physical Therapy, 1997; 77(4): 354-60.	171 consecutive LBP patients, w/ or w/o leg pain presenting at 5 clinics. Duration: 14 days to 2 yrs.	Patients all assessed with McKenzie methods and Waddell signs tested. Patients classified and treated over 30 days. 6-mon phone follow-up to determine work status as only outcome.	Centralization occurred in 73%. Low Waddell scores in 83%. Centralizers returned to work more frequently than non-centralizers (p=.038). High Waddell scores overrode centralization as a predictor. There was a complex relationship between centralization and Waddell scores re. RTW.	The probability of RTW is greater if a patient centralizes. Waddell tests should be performed even with centralizers.
Sufka A, Hauger B, Trenary M, et al. **Centralization of low back pain and perceived functional outcome.** Journal of Orthopedics and Sports Physical Therapy, 1998. 27(3): 205-12.	36 LBP patients w/ or w/o leg pain. Pain duration: QTF1: 6, QTF2: 15, QTF3: 15 Pain location: QTF1: 15 (back pain only), QTF2: 7, QTF3: 14 (below knee)	All patients evaluated with McKenzie methods. Treatment based on McK assessment findings. Outcomes: Oswestry, Spinal Function Sort at baseline and 14-day FU.	94% agreement/interrater reliability w/ centralization in pilot group Complete centralization occurred in 69% of patients over 14 days (mean=4.3) Acute=83%, subacute=73% & chronic=60% / QTF1=80%, QTF2-73% QTF3=43% Fewer chronics and fewer w/ pain below the knee completely centralized.	LBP sufferers show greater improvement (functional outcomes) when there is evidence of "complete" centralization within 14 days than when there is not. Time of complete centralization was no longer for chronics or those with pain below the knee.
Werneke M, Hart D, Cook D. **A descriptive study of the centralization phenomenon: a prospective analysis.** Spine, 1999. 24: 676-83.	289 consecutive patients with acute neck or LBP w/ or w/o referred spinal sxs referred to PhysTher.	Subjects assessed & cate-gorized into 3 pain pattern grps using McK assessm't. Pain location & intensity, funct'l status, # treatm't visits compared between the 3 grps.	Reliability between judges: excellent for distal pain location and categorizing. Cent'zers-31%, partial cent'zers-46%, non-cent'zers- 23%. Cent'zers had sign'tly fewer visits (p<0.001), less pain intensity and better function (p<0.001) than other grps	Categorization by changes, or lack of changes, in pain location to mechanical assessment allowed identification of patients with improved outcomes and facilitated treatment planning or those in need of more extensive evaluations.

Study	Participants	Design/Methods	Results	Conclusions
Werneke M, Hart D, Cook D **Centralization phenomenon as a prognostic factor for chronic low back pain and disability** Spine, 2001. 26:758-65	225 consecutive pts. with acute neck or LBP w/ or w/o referred spinal sxs. 73% were WC.	Pts. underwent mechanical assessment and categorized into those whose pain centralized and those who did not. Treatment was individualized and based on McK methods. 22 independent variables assessed with five dependent variables at 12 months post-discharge.	Pain pattern classification was a predictor of future pain, return to work, activity interference, and continued use of health care. Perceived disability predicted only activity interference while work satisfaction predicted only pain intensity. No variable predicted sick leave at work.	These results support that physical factors are important predictors of chronic LBP and disability. Identifying those whose pain does not centralize is an important predictor of future disability and healthcare usage.
Donelson R, Plante D, Likosky D, Orgren R, Lindstrom U Patients' Low Back Pain "Experience": A Natural History Survey Unpublished; Presented at the 2001 annual meeting of the Dartmouth/Northern New England Primary Care Cooperative Research Network	349 consecutive LBP patients presenting for care to 15 primary care, physical therapy, chiropractic, and spine surgical practices completed a 49-question, self-administered, written survey.	The survey targeted pts' experience with recurrences, some of their episode characteristics, changes in pain location during episodes, and how pain is affected by various positions and activities.	64% of patients had had previous episodes. 54% said their recent episodes were worse than their initial episodes in 3 of 5 "worsening" variables. 80% said their pain changed locations during episodes; 57% said their pain moved distally during episode progression and then proximally during recovery. Positions and activities requiring lumbar flexion significantly aggravated subjects' pain far more than being erect or recumbent (p<0.0001).	These findings support the value of seeking better understanding of specific characteristics of LBP in order to determine how patients so often cause and then recover from episodes as well as progress from acute self-limiting episodes to prolonged, chronic, and more complex problems.
Werneke M, Hart D Categorizing patients with occupational low back pain by use of the Quebec Task Force classification system versus pain pattern classification procedures: discriminant and predictive validity Physical Therapy, 2004. 84:243-54.	171 pts with acute work-related low back pain referred for physical therapy were analyzed.	Pts completed pain and psychosocial questionnaires at initial examination and discharge and pain diagrams throughout intervention. Pts classified patients using Quebec Task Force and MDT pain pattern classifications at intake.	QTFC and MDT pain data could be used to differentiate patients by pain intensity or disability at intake, however intake pain classification predicted pain intensity, disability, and work status at discharge, but QTFC did not.	Evidence of predictive validity of the MDT pain data at intake.

Study	Participants	Design/Methods	Results	Conclusions
Aina S, May S, Clare H **The centralization phenomenon of spinal symptoms - a systematic review** Manual Therapy, 2004, 9:134-43	Fourteen studies identified and reviewed	Systematic review; selection criteria determined prior to computer-aided literature search. Data extracted by two independent reviewers with disagreements resolved by third reviewer. Quality of studies varied.	Centralization prevalence rate of was 70% in 731 sub-acute back patients, 52% in 325 chronic LBP patients. Centralization can be reliably determined (kappa values 0.51–1.0) and was consistently associated with good outcomes. Failure to centralize associated with poor outcomes.	Centralization identifies a substantial subgroup of spinal patients; it can be reliably detected and is associated with a good prognosis. Centralization evaluation should take place and then monitored in spinal pain patients.
Rasmussen C, Nielsen G, Hansen V, Jensen O, Schioettz-Christensen B **Rates of lumbar disc surgery before and after implementation of multidisciplinary nonsurgical spine clinics.** Spine, 2005. 30: p. 2469-73.	In North Jutland County, Denmark (500,000 population). In 1997, two non-surgical spine clinics established focused on MDT care and educational program for general doctors for pts with 1 to 3 months' of sciatica, with or without low back pain.	Data on rates of lumbar disc surgery were obtained from the National Registry of Patients over the next four years.	The annual rate of lumbar disc operations for pts in N. Jutland County decreased from 60-80 per 100,000 before 1997 to 40 per 100,000 in 2001 (P = 0.00), and the rate of elective, first-time disc surgeries decreased by approximately two thirds (P = 0.00). The rate of lumbar disc operations in the rest of Denmark remained unchanged during the same period.	The implementation of these non-surgical spine clinics coincided closely with a significant reduction in the rate of lumbar disc surgery. The observed reduction seems most likely to be causally associated with educational activities and improved patient care provided by the clinics.
Skytte L, May S, Petersen P **Centralization - its prognostic value in patients with referred symptoms and sciatica.** Spine, 2005. 30:E(293-9)	104 consecutive patients referred for investigation of possible disc herniation.	60 recruited underwent a standardized MDT evaluation to expose 2 groups: central'n (CG) and non-central'n group (NCG). All patients were treated in the same way and were followed for one year. If patients did not have improvement surgery was considered. Outcomes included back and leg pain, disability, Nottingham Health Profile, and surgical outcome.	25 patients were classified in the CG, 35 were NCG and other baseline characteristics were similar between groups. At 1, 2, and 3 months, the CG had significantly better outcomes than the NCG. At 2 months, the CG had more improvements in leg pain (P < 0.007), disability (P < 0.001), and Nottingham Health Profile (P < 0.001). After 1 year, disability was less in the CG (P < 0.029). 3 CG patients underwent surgery vs. 16 NCG (P < 0.01). The odds ratio for surgery in the NCG was 6.2.	Patients with sciatica and suspected disc herniation who have a centralization response will have significantly better outcomes. Patients who do not have a centralization will be 6 times more likely to undergo surgery.

Randomized Clinical Trials: Black Box Directional Interventions
(RCTs demonstrating the benefits of lumbar extension and/or the aggravation of flexion)

Study	Participants	Design/Methods	Results	Conclusions
Donelson R, Grant W, Kamps C, Medcalf R Pain response to sagittal end-range spinal motion. A prospective, randomized, multi-centered trial Spine 16: S206-12, 1991	145 pts. with LBP with or without leg pain presenting to 12 different PT practices for care	All pts. underwent a scripted assessment protocol of standing and recumbent repeated end-range lumbar testing in flexion and extension while monitoring symptom intensity and location response with VAS and pain drawings. Pts were randomized to either performing extension tests first vs. flexion tests first.	It made no difference in pain response whether flexion or extension tests were performed first. Overall, 40% centralized/ abolished their pain with extension while worsening worsened with flexion; only 7% centralized/abolished their pain with flexion and worsened with extension. No subject's pain improved in both directions.	It made no difference in what order directional testing in the sagittal plane was performed. With scripted testing only in the sagittal plane, both a "directional preference" & "vulnerability" were identified in 47%.
Williams M, Hawley J, McKenzie R, Van Wijmen P **A comparison of the effects of two sitting postures on back and referred pain** Spine, 1991. 16(10): 1185-91.	210 patients with low back and/or referred pain presenting for care to PTs.	Subjects randomly assigned to either a kyphotic posture or lordotic posture (using a lumbar roll for support) for 24-48 hrs. Pain location, back pain and leg pain intensity were assessed.	Lordotic sitting reduced back and leg pain intensity significantly more than did kyphotic sitting and let to referred pain shifting toward the back (centralization).	Lordotic sitting resulted in reductions in back and leg pain and centralization of pain.
Spratt K, Weinstein J, Lehmann T, Woody J, Sayre H **Efficacy of flexion and extension treatments incorporating braces for low-back pain patients with retrodisplacement, spondylo listhesis, or normal sagittal translation** Spine 18:1839-49, 1993	56 patients with low-back pain with either "normal" translation, retrodisplacement or spondylolisthesis	Patients randomized to either flexion or extension treatment (consisting of a directional brace and exercises and an audio-slide presentation favoring the assigned direction of care), or a control with an abdominal wrap without exercise and a general audio-slide program. One month follow-up: compliance, ROM, strength, VAS, Million pain interference, pt. satisfaction	18% considered non-compliant with 80% in the flexion group with 75% of those "spondys". Bracing did not decrease ROM. Across all 3 diagnostic groups, flexion treatment resulted in low benefits while extension treatment resulted in relatively large benefits.	The response to extension bracing and exercise was significantly better that flexion or the control. The authors hypothesized that, since all 3 diagnostic groups benefited from extension, radiographic instability might more appropriately be considered a corroborative sign of advanced discogenic problems that responded well to extension treatment.

Study	Participants	Design/Methods	Results	Conclusions
Snook S, Webster B, McGorry R, Fogleman, M, McCann, K **The reduction of chronic non-specific low back pain through the control of early morning flexion: a randomized controlled trial** Spine 23:2601-7, 1998	86 volunteers with chronic or recurrent LBP, not under current care, no hx of surgery, non-WC, not pregnant	No intervention first 6 mons: base-line pain diarying; then randomized to 6 mons of either instruction in the elimination of early morning flexion (based on theory that the IV disc is a common source of chronic LBP-internal disc disruption and is vulnerable to early morning flexion) or a sham treatment of six common exercises (Phase 1); then sham crossed to flexion avoidance last 6 mon (Phase 2). Diaries kept daily re. pain intensity, activity interference, & medication use.	Signif't pain reduction (p<0.01), reduction of meds (p<0.05) and impairment (p<0.01) in the flexion avoidance groups in both Phase 1 and 2 for AM avoidance group. There was an 18% decrease in pain-days/mon. 80% intended to continue to voluntarily restrict AM flexion	Avoidance of morning flexion resulted in highly significant reduction in pain, impairment and the use of meds. This gives support to the theory that low back pain is discogenic. Subjects recognized the relationship between their improvement and the avoidance of morning flexion.
Snook S, Webster B, McGorry R, Fogleman M, McCann K The reduction of chronic non-specific low back pain through the control of early morning lumbar flexion: a randomized controlled trial: a 3-year follow-up Unpublished: presented at N.Amer McK Conference, June 2000	As above	Follow-up 3 yrs. after study completion – 4 years from initial intervention.	83% response rate. 62% still voluntarily restricting AM flexion. 74% reported further reductions in pain-days/mon, 22% reported increases and 2% the same. In total, there was another 46% decrease in pain-days/mon. to add to the original 18% (56% decrease overall).	A high percentage of subjects voluntarily continued with AM flexion avoidance strategies resulting in even further improvements in pain control over three years.

Study	Participants	Design/Methods	Results	Conclusions
Larsen K, Weidick F, Leboeuf-Yde C **Can passive prone extensions of the back prevent back problems? A randomized, controlled intervention trial of 314 military conscripts.** Spine, 2002. 27: p. 2747-52.	249 healthy Danish male conscripts entering their basic military training.	Conscripts randomized into two groups: intervention and no intervention (8 mon. of basic military training). Intervention group received one 40-minute lesson on back problems, posture and ergonomics and had to perform passive prone extensions of the back daily during 8 months of their military training. Data collected through questionnaires at the start of military duty and after 10 months. Outcome variables: self-reported back pain in last 3 weeks and last yr.; physician consultations for LBP during their military service.	In intention-to-treat analysis, significantly fewer persons in the intervention group versus those in control group reported back problems during the last year (33% versus 51%). Significantly fewer persons in the intervention group versus those in the control group consulted the regiment infirmary (9% versus 25%). Most differences were in subjects with history of LBP vs. no history.	It is possible to reduce the prevalence of LBP and the use of health care services during military service using passive prone lumbar extension exercises based on the theory of the disc as a pain generator and ergonomic instructions. Prevention for subjects with prior LBP history was significant vs. those with no history.
Long et al Spine, 2004. 29:2593-2602.	SEE PAIN RESPONSE -RELATED RCTS			

Pain Response Randomized Clinical Trials and Systematic Reviews

Study	Participants	Design/Methods	Results	Conclusions
Delitto A, Cibulka M, Erhard R, Bowling R, Tenhula, J **Evidence for an extension-mobilization category in acute low back syndrome: a prescriptive validation pilot study** Physical Therapy, 1993. 73(4):216-28.	Of a total of 39 patients with low back syndrome (LBS) referred for physical therapy, 24 patients were classified as having signs (centralization) and symptoms indicating treatment with an extension-mobilization approach. The remaining subjects were dismissed from the study.	Patients in the extension-mobilization category were randomly assigned to either mobilization and extension (a treatment matching their category) (n=14) or a flexion exercise regimen (an unmatched treatment) (n=10). Outcomes: modified Oswestry LBP Questionnaire at baseline, at 3 and 5 days after initiation of treatment.	Subjects treated with extension and mobilization positively responded at a faster rate than did those treated with a flexion-oriented program.	A priori classification of selected patients with LBS into a treatment category of extension and mobilization and subsequently treating the patients with specified interventions can be an effective approach to conservative management of selected patients.

Study	Participants	Design/Methods	Results	Conclusions
Fritz J, Delitto A, and Erhard R **Comparison of classification-based physical therapy with therapy based on clinical practice guidelines for patients with acute low back pain: a randomized clinical trial** Spine, 2003. 28(13):1363-71.	78 subjects with work-related low back pain of less than 3 weeks duration. Evaluated and classified into Delitto categories, including central'n/ specific exercise subgroup.	Pts. randomized to receive therapy determined by their baseline classification or therapy based on the Agency for Health Care Policy and Research guidelines. Subjects followed for 1 year. Outcomes: impairment index, Oswestry scale, SF-36 component scores, satisfaction, medical costs, and return to work status.	After four weeks, subjects receiving classification-based therapy showed greater change on the Oswestry (P = 0.023) and the SF-36 physical component (P = 0.029), pt. satisfaction (P = 0.006) and return to full-duty work status (P = 0.017). After 1 year, there was a trend toward reduced Oswestry scores in the classification-based group (P = 0.063). Median total medical costs for 1 year were lower in classification-based group (P = 0.13 ($774 vs. $1004)	For patients with acute, work-related low back pain, the use of a classification-based approach resulted in improved disability and return to work status after 4 weeks, as compared with therapy based on clinical practice guidelines. Further research is needed on the optimal timing and methods of intervention for patients with acute low back pain.
Schenk R, Jazefczyk C, Kopf A **A randomized trial comparing interventions in patients with lumbar posterior derangement** J. of Manip & Physio'l Therap'cs, 2003. 11:95-102.	25 pts. referred to P.T. for treatment of their lumbar radiculopathy who were classified as a McKenzie "derangement" upon initial examination.	Pts. randomized to either spinal mobilization or therapeutic exercise acc. to McKenzie methods. All seen for 3 P.T. visits; Pain and function (Oswestry) measured at baseline and discharge.	Therapeutic exercise produced significantly greater decrease in pain level (p<.01) and greater improvement in function (p<.03) compared to the mobilization group.	Exercises selected by repeated movement testing created greater pain reduction and recovery of function than joint mobilization in acute lumbar derangements. Repeated movements as part of the lumbar evaluation may be important.

Study	Participants	Design/Methods	Results	Conclusions
Long A, Donelson R, Fung T **Does it matter which exercise? A randomized controlled trial of exercise for low back pain** Spine, 2004. 29:2593-2602.	312 consecutive LBP pts with or without leg pain, no or one neurologic sign, acute, subacute, or chronic, referred to one of 11 PT clinics. Underwent MDT assessment by Credentialed PTs to identify those with a directional preference (DP): extension, flexion or lateral.	DP pts randomized to exercises that Matched or were opposite to their DP (Opp), or were non-directional (ND). All given activity advice, rationale for their exercise and education to minimize fear-avoidance behaviors. Outcomes collected at baseline and two weeks. Primary outcome measures: back and leg pain intensity. Secondary measures: patient satisfaction, Quebec Task Force severity class, medication use, the Beck Depression Inventory, interference with work and leisure activity, and the Roland-Morris Disability Questionnaire.	40% out of work due to LBP, 13% acute, 32% subacute, and 55% chronic. 47% had back pain only, 18% referred pain above the knee, 17% below the knee, and 17% had one positive neurologic sign. 74% had DP, 83% preferring extension, 7% flexion, 10% lateral. Only one pt. in Matched group withdrew due to worsening symptoms compared vs. 43% in Opp group and 20% in ND group. 95% of Matched group reported either Better or Resolved and no one Worse, vs. only 23% Better or Resolved in the Opp group and 42% in the ND group. In both Opp and ND groups, 15% reported being worse (despite having a DP at baseline. All 7 secondary outcomes were significantly better in the Matched group than either Opp or ND.	It matters which exercise is prescribed in the large DP subgroup of LBP. Effective, ineffective, and even counter-productive exercises were identified. Improving or eliminating pts' pain significantly decreased medication use and improved all six secondary outcome measures. Due to attrition in Opp and ND groups, this study could not continue past 2 wks of follow-up.
Brennan GP, Fritz JM, Hunter SJ, Thackeray A, Delitto A, Erhard R **Identifying subgroups of patients with acute/ subacute "nonspecific" low back pain. Results of a randomized clinical trial** Spine 2006, 31:623-31	123 pts with < 90d of LBP, with and without referred pain, referred to P.T. for treatment. Excluded: lateral or kyphotic deformity, signs of nerve root compression. Pts classified into 1 of 3 treatment categories based on treatment expected to be beneficial.	RCT; After classification, pts. randomized to manipulation, stabilization exercise, specific directional exercise.	Patients receiving treatments matching their category experienced greater short- and long-term reductions in disability than those receiving unmatched treatments.	Nonspecific low back pain should not be viewed as a homogenous condition. Outcomes can be improved when subgrouping is used to guide treatment decision-making.

Study	Participants	Design/Methods	Results	Conclusions
Browder DA, Childs JD, Cleland JA, Fritz, J **Effectiveness of an extension-oriented treatment approach in a subgroup of patients with low back pain: a randomized clinical trial** Subm'd for publ'n; McKenzie Conf. of the Americas, 2006, Montreal	Acute LBP patients with pain distal to the buttocks and centralization identified at baseline examination	RCT; subjects randomized to either extension-oriented treatment or stabilization exercises. Outcome measures gathered at 1 week, 4 weeks, and 6 months.	Extension-oriented treatment significantly better at one week, 4 weeks, and 6 months.	Developing treatment-based subgrouping procedures for patients with LBP is an important priority. Validity of any subgroup is ultimately determined by treatment outcomes. Directional preference and centralization appear to be important sub-grouping criteria
Clare H, Adams R, Maher C **A systematic review of efficacy of McKenzie therapy for spinal pain.** Australian Journal of Physiotherapy, 2004. 50: p. 209-16.	Databases searched: DARE, CINAHL, CENTRAL, EMBASE, MEDLINE and PEDro.	A systematic review of RCTs of trials providing treatment according to McK principles reporting on one of the following: pain, disability, quality of life, work status, global perceived effect, medication use, health care contacts, or recurrence.	Six eligible trials compared McK therapy to a comparison treatment: NSAIDS, educational booklet, back massage and back care advice, strength training, and spinal mobilization and general exercises. At short term: McK provided a mean 8.6 point greater pain reduction on 0-100 scale and a 5.4 greater reduction in disability on 0-100 scaled than comparison. At intermediate follow-up: relative risk of work absence = 0.81 (0.46 to 1.44) favoring McK, however the comparison treatments provided a 1.2 point greater disability reduction (95% CI -2.0 to 4.5). In the one cervical trial, McKenzie therapy provided similar benefits to an exercise program.	For LBP patients, McK therapy provides a greater decrease in pain and disability in the short term than other standard therapies. Making a firm conclusion at this time on LBP treatment effectiveness is difficult because there are insufficient data on long term effects on outcomes other than pain and disability and no trial has yet compared McKenzie to placebo or no treatment. There are also insufficient data available on neck pain patients.
Cook C, Hegedus E, Ramey **Physical therapy exercise intervention based on classification using the patent response method: a systematic review of the literature** J. of Manipulative & Physiologic Therapeutics, 2005, 13:152-62	82 pain response classification studies reviewed	Systematic review using Pedro scale for measuring quality of design.	Five studies met standards for high quality. Four demonstrated superior outcomes using exercise therapy based on a patient-response method of classification (Delitto, Fritz, Long, Schenk). Fifth study reported exercise to be less effective than manipulation (Erhard).	Exercise leads to improved outcomes in patients classified according to patient-response methods. The evidence for the value of including a centralization evaluation as a classification criterion is quite compelling. This form of classification reliably differentiates discogenic from non-discogenic symptoms.

Studies correlating pain response patterns with symptomatic disc pathology

Study	Participants	Design/Methods	Results	Conclusions
Kopp J, Alexander H, Turocy R, Levrini M, Lichtman D The use of lumbar extension in the evaluation and treatment of patients with acute herniated nucleus pulposus: a preliminary report Clinical Orthopedics 202:211-8, 1986	67 pts. admitted for care of acute LBP radiating to calf or foot, at least one significant sign of nerve root compression, limited lumbar extension, no non-disc etiologies, sx severity precluding outpt management or failure to improve after 6 wks of conservative care. Excluded if lumbar extension testing increased leg pain.	Retrospective review of study cohort. Pts directed in progressive extension positioning/exercising. Patients grouped by their response to treatment as 1-responders and 2-those requiring surgery. Responders discharged from hospital, neural signs resolved, elimination of pain distal to the knee, return to normal activity.	35 pts. (52%) responded to extension treatment. 34 achieved normal extension, most within 1-3 days, all but one within 5 days. 32 pts. underwent CT scans and underwent disc surgery (56% free fragments, 19% swollen or displaced nerve roots, 19% bulging discs, 6% no description).	52% of pts with LB, leg pain & neurologic signs rapidly regained extension ROM, eliminated their pain, and recovered, many after prolonged outpatient treatment. Those who did not respond to extension required surgery with a high incidence of free fragments and nerve root displacement.
Donelson R, Silva G, Murphy K. The centralization phenomenon: its usefulness in evaluating and treating referred pain Spine, 1990. 15(3): 211-13.	87 patients with LBP and radiating leg pain presenting to a general orthopedic practice. Pain duration: 53 acutes (0-4 wks), 15 subacutes (4-12 wks), 19 chronics (12+ wks.)	Independent retrospective chart review. Patients all assessed and/or treated with MDT form of care. Presence or absence of centralization on initial assessment correlated with treatment outcomes. Outcomes only at time of discharge: pain relief, return to activity/work, patient satisfaction.	Centralization occurred in 87% of all patients (89/87/84% of acutes, subacutes, chronics). 98/77/81% of centralizers, 17/50/33% of non-centralizers had good or excellent outcomes. Only 4 surgical disc patients: all non-centralizers, all did well with surgery.	Centralization occurred commonly and its presence or absence was a strong predictor of treatment outcome and the presence or absence of surgical disc pathology.
Donelson R, Aprill R, Medcalf R, Grant W A prospective study of centralization of lumbar and referred pain Spine 22: 1115-22, 1997	63 pts with LBP and varying degrees of leg pain and altered sensation referred for lumbar discography due to pain sufficiently severe to warrant invasive testing, failure of conservative care, and 1 or more MRI studies w/o compelling surgical findings	Consecutive discography pts. first underwent MDT assessment and classified as centralizers, peripheralizers, or no effect on pain. Routine lumbar discography and CT imaging followed. Outcomes of the two types of assessment were compared.	50% centralized, 25% peripheralized only, and 25% reported no effect on their leg pain with the MDT evaluation. 57% had positive discograms of which 81% did not leak. 43% were negative. 74% of centralizers, 69% of peripheralizers and only 12% of no effect pts had pos. discograms. 91% of centralizers had intact annuli but only 54% of peripheralizers.	Despite the chronicity of the pts, 50% still demonstrated a reversibility of their pathology, which was shown in 74% of cases to be disc. The ability to distinguish between a pos. and neg. discogram based on MDT findings was highly significant (p<0.001).

Study	Participants	Design/Methods	Results	Conclusions
Snook S, Webster B, McGorry R, Fogleman, M, McCann, K **The reduction of chronic non-specific low back pain through the control of early morning flexion: a randomized controlled trial** Spine 23:2601-7, 1998	86 volunteers with chronic or recurrent LBP, not under current care, no hx of surgery, non-WC, not pregnant	No intervention first 6 mons (baseline pain diarying); then randomized to 6 mons of either instruction in **the elimination of early morning flexion (based on theory that the IV disc is a common source of chronic LBP-internal disc disruption and is vulnerable to early morning flexion)** or a sham treatment of six common exercises (Phase 1); then sham crossed to flexion avoidance last 6 mon (Phase 2). Diaries kept daily re. pain intensity, activity interference, & medication use.	Significant pain reduction (p<0.01), reduction of meds (p<0.05), and impairment (p<0.01) in the flexion avoidance groups at both Phase 1 and 2 for AM avoidance group. There was an 18% decrease in pain-days/mon. 80% intended to continue to voluntarily restrict AM flexion	Avoidance of morning flexion resulted in highly significant reduction in pain, impairment and the use of meds. This gives support to the theory that low back pain is disco-genic. Subjects recognized the relationship between their improvement and the avoidance of morning flexion.
Laslett M, Öberg B, Aprill C, McDonald B **Centralization as a predictor of provocation discography results in chronic low back pain, and the influence of disability and distress on diagnostic power.** The Spine Journal, 2005. 5:370-80.	107 consecutive pts with persistent LBP referred by for interventional radiological diagnostic procedures. Pts were typically disabled and displayed high levels of psychosocial distress, failed conservative therapies, including pts. with previous lumbar surgery.	A prospective, blinded, concurrent, reference standard-related validity design. Patients received a single physical therapy examination, followed by lumbar provocation discography at 2 or more levels. Sensitivity, specificity, and likelihood ratios of the centralization phenomenon were analyzed in the full group and in subgroups defined by psychometric measures. Index test: centralization Other variables: psychometric eval: Roland–Morris, Zung, Modified Somatic Perception questionnaires, Distress Risk Assessment Method, and visual analog scale for pain intensity.	38 could not tolerate a full physical examination and were excluded from the main analysis. Disability and pain intensity ratings were high, and distress was common. Sensitivity, specificity, and positive likelihood ratios for centralization were 40%, 94%, and 6.9 respectively. In those with severe disability, sensitivity, specificity, and positive likelihood ratios were 46%, 80%, 3.2. In those with distress, 45%, 89%, 4.1. In those with moderate, minimal, or no disability, sensitivity and specificity were 37% and 100% and for no or minimal distress 35% and 100%.	Centralization is highly specific to positive discography but specificity is reduced in the presence of severe disability or psycho-social distress.

Study	Participants	Design/Methods	Results	Conclusions
Skytte L, May S, Petersen P **Centralization - its prognostic value in patients with referred symptoms and sciatica.** Spine, 2005. 30:E(293-9)	104 consecutive patients referred for investigation of possible disc herniation.	60 recruited underwent a standardized MDT evaluation to expose 2 groups: central'n (CG) and noncentral'n group (NCG). All patients were treated in the same way and were followed for one year. If patients did not have improvement surgery was considered. Outcomes included back and leg pain, disability, Nottingham Health Profile, and surgical outcome.	25 patients were classified in the CG, 35 were NCG and other baseline characteristics were similar between groups. At 1, 2, and 3 months, the CG had significantly better outcomes than the NCG. At 2 months, the CG had more improvements in leg pain (P < 0.007), disability (P < 0.001), and Nottingham Health Profile (P < 0.001). After 1 year, disability was less in the CG (P < 0.029). 3 CG patients underwent surgery vs. 16 NCG (P < 0.01). The odds ratio for surgery in the NCG was 6.2.	Patients with sciatica and suspected disc herniation who have a centralization response will have significantly better outcomes. Patients who do not have centralization will be 6 times more likely to undergo surgery.
Rasmussen C, Nielsen G, Hansen V, Jensen O, Schioettz-Christensen B **Rates of lumbar disc surgery before and after implementation of multidisciplinary nonsurgical spine clinics.** Spine, 2005. 30: p. 2469-73.	In North Jutland County, Denmark (500,000 population). In 1997, two non-surgical spine clinics established focused on MDT care and educational program for general doctors for pts with 1 to 3 months' of sciatica, with or without low back pain.	Data on rates of lumbar disc surgery were obtained from the National Registry of Patients over the next four years.	The annual rate of lumbar disc operations for pts in N. Jutland County decreased from 60-80 per 100,000 before 1997 to 40 per 100,000 in 2001 (P = 0.00), and the rate of elective, first-time disc surgeries decreased by approximately two thirds (P = 0.00). The rate of lumbar disc operations in the rest of Denmark remained unchanged during the same period.	The implementation of these non-surgical spine clinics coincided closely with a significant reduction in the rate of lumbar disc surgery. The observed reduction seems most likely to be causally associated with educational activities and improved patient care provided by the clinics.
Long A, Donelson R, Fung T **Acute or chronic back pain or sciatica: Is differentiation always necessary?** Submitted for publication	312 consecutively seen LBP-only patients, with or without sciatica, and of all durations, were assessed using MDT methods. 230 (74%) found to have a directional preference (DP). 80 randomized to MDT care with directionally-matched exercises were this study's subjects.	Secondary analysis (ANOVA) to determine outcome differences by duration and pain location/ severity. Outcomes included back/leg pain intensity, medication use, activity interference, self-rated improvement, Roland-Morris Disability Questionnaire (RMDQ), and Beck Depression Inventory.	When treated with DP-concordant exercises, DP subjects reported significant improvement in every outcome measure (p<.001) independent of duration or pain location/severity subgroups. Acute DP subjects reported the greatest improvement in LBP (p=.036) and RMDQ scores (p=.026).	Regardless of pain duration or location (including sciatica), DP subjects substantially decreased pain intensity and improved every secondary outcome measure using concordant directional exercises. DP may reflect a pain-generator with mechan'l characteristics and symptom responses to MDT loading tests that span a broad spectrum of LBP.

References

1. Abelson R and Petersen M, *An operation to ease back pain bolsters the bottom line, too*, in *New York Times*. 2003: New York, NY. p. 1.
2. Adams M and Hutton W, *Gradual disc prolapse*. Spine, 1985. 10: p. 524-531.
3. Adams MA, et al., *Effects of backward bending on lumbar intervertebral discs. Relevance to physical therapy treatments for low back pain*. Spine, 2000. 25(4): p. 431-7; discussion 438.
4. Aina S, May S, and Clare H, *The centralization phenomenon of spinal symptoms - a systematic review*. Manual Therapy, 2004. 9: p. 134-43.
5. Alexander A, Jones A, and Rosenbaum D, *Nonoperative management of herniated nucleus pulposus: patient selection by the extension sign; long-term follow-up*. Orthopedic Review, 1992. 21(2): p. 181-8.
6. Andersson G, *The epidemiology of spinal disorders*, in *The Adult Spine*, J. Frymoyer, Editor. 1997, Lippincott - Raven: Philadelphia - New York. p. 93-141.
7. Andersson G, et al., *Summary statement: treatment of the painful motion segment*. Spine, 2005. 30(16S): p. S1.
8. Andersson G, Svensson H-O, and Oden A, *The intensity of work recovery in low back pain*. Spine, 1983. 8: p. 880-4.
9. Battie M, et al., *Managing low back pain: attitudes and treatment preferences of physicial therapists*. Physical Therapy, 1994. 74(3): p. 219-226.
10. Bigos S, et al., *Acute low back problems in adults: clinical practice guidelines, quick reference guide no. 14*. 1994, U.S. Department of Health and Human Services, Agency for Health Care Policy and Research: Rockville, MD.
11. Boden S, Davis D, and Dina T, *Abnormal magnetic-resonance scans of the lumbar spine in asymptomatic subjects: a prospective investigation*. Journal of Bone and Joint Surgery, 1990. 72: p. 403-8.
12. Boos N, et al., *The diagnostic accuracy of magnetic resonance imaging, work perception, and psychosocial factors in identifying symptomatic disc herniations*. Spine, 1995. 20(24): p. 2613-25.
13. Borkan J. *Are we stuck?* in *International Forum for Primary Care Research in Low Back Pain*. 2004. Edmonton, Alberta, Canada.
14. Borkan J, et al., *A report from the second international forum for primary care research on low back pain: reexamining priorities*. Spine, 1998. 23(18): p. 1992-6.
15. Bouter L, Pennick V, and Bombardier C, *Cochrane back review group*. Spine, 2003. 28(12): p. 1215-8.
16. Bouter L, van Tulder M, and Koes B, *Methodologic issues in low back pain research in primary care*. Spine, 1998. 23(18): p. 2014-20.
17. Brennan G, et al., *Identifying subgroups of patients with acute/subacute "nonspecific" low back pain. Results of a randomized clinical trial*. Spine, 2006. 31: p. 623-31.
18. Browder D, et al. *Effectiveness of an extension-oriented treatment approach in a subgroup of patients with low back pain: a randomized clinical trial*. in *2006 McKenzie Conference of the Americas*. 2006. Montreal, Quebec.
19. Buchbinder R, Jolley D, and Wyatt M, *Population based intervention to change back pain beliefs and disability: three part evaluation*. British Medical Journal, 2001. 322: p. 1516-20.
20. Burstein A, *Do they work and are they useful?* Journal of Bone and Joint Surgery, 1993. 75-A: p. 1743-4.
21. Burton A, et al., *European guidelines for prevention in low back pain*. 2004.

22. Carey J, *Medical guesswork: from heart surgery to prostrate care, the health industry knows little about which common treatments really work*, in *BusinessWeek*. 2006. p. 73-9.

23. Carey T, et al., *The outcomes and costs of care for acute low back pain among patients seen by primary care practitioners, chiropractors, and orthopedic surgeons.* New England Journal of Medicine, 1995. 333(14): p. 913-7.

24. Chavennes A, et al., *Acute low back pain: patients' perceptions of pain four weeks after initial diagnosis and treatment in general practice.* 1986. 36: p. 271-3.

25. Cherkin D, et al., *A comparison of physical therapy, chiropractic manipulation, and provision of an educational booklet for the treatment of patients with low back pain.* New England Journal of Medicine, 1998. 339: p. 1021-29.

26. Cherkin D, et al., *Predicting poor outcomes for back pain seen in primary care using patients' own criteria.* Spine, 1996. 21: p. 2900-2907.

27. Cherkin D, et al., *Physician variation in diagnostic testing for low back pain: who you see is what you get.* Arthritis and Rheumatism, 1994. 37(1): p. 15-22.

28. Childs J, et al., *A clinical prediction rule to identify patients with low back pain most likely to benefit from spinal manipulation: a validation study.* Annals of Internal Medicine, 2004. 141: p. 920-8.

29. Churchill W. *Radio speech.* 1939.

30. Clare H, Adams R, and Maher C, *Reliability of McKenzie classification of patients with cervical and lumbar pain.* Journal of Manipulative and Physiological Therapeutics, 2005. 28(2): p. 122-7.

31. Clare H, Adams R, and Maher C, *Reliability of the McKenzie spinal pain classification using patient assessment forms.* Physiotherapy, 2004. 90: p. 114-9.

32. Cook C, Hegedus E, and Ramey K, *Physical therapy exercise intervention based on classification using the patent response method: a systematic review of the literature.* Journal of Manipulative and Physiological Therapeutics, 2005. 13: p. 152-62.

33. Corp NZAC, *New Zealand Accident Compensation Corp Chronic Backs Study.* 1994, New Zealand Accident Compensation Corp: Auckland, New Zealand.

34. Croft P, et al., *Low back pain in the community and in hospitals.* 1994, The Arthritis and Rheumatism Council, Epidemiology Research Unit And The Rheumatic Diseases Center, University of Manchester: Manchester, UK. p. 1-33.

35. Croft P, et al., *Outcome of low back pain in general practice: a prospective study.* British Medical Journal, 1998. 316: p. 1356-9.

36. Delitto A, *Research in low back pain: time to stop seeking the elusive "magic bullet".* Journal of the American Physical Therapy Association, 2005. 85.

37. Delitto A, et al., *Evidence for an extension-mobilization category in acute low back syndrome: a prescriptive validation pilot study.* Physical Therapy, 1993. 73(4): p. 216-28.

38. Delitto A, Erhard R, and Bowling R, *A treatment-based classification approach to low back syndrome: identifying and staging patients for conservative management.* Physical Therapy, 1995. 75: p. 470-89.

39. Deyo R and Weinstein J, *Primary care: low back pain.* New England Journal of Medicine, 2001. 344(5): p. 363-70.

40. Dillane J, Fry J, and Kalton G, *Acute back syndrome: a study from general practice.* British Medical Journal, 1966. 2: p. 82-4.

41. Dixon A, *Progress and problems in low back pain research.* Rheumatologic Rehabilitation, 1973. 12(4): p. 165-75.

42. Donelson R, *Conservative care of the low back: the McKenzie approach*, in *Conservative Care of Low Back Pain*, R.A. AH White, Editor. 1990, Williams & Wilkins. p. 97-105.

43. Donelson R. *Do meaningful low back pain subgroups exist and how can they be identified?* in *Fifth International Forum for the Primary Care Research in Low Back Pain.* 2002. Montreal, Quebec.

44. Donelson R, *Evidence-based low back pain classification: Improving care at its foundation.* Europa Medicophysica, 2004. 40: p. 37-40.
45. Donelson R, *Managing low back pain: the initial evaluation. Mechanical assessment simplifies the assessment process and points to appropriate therapy.* Journal of Musculoskeletal Medicine, 2004.
46. Donelson R, *The McKenzie approach to evaluating and treating low back pain.* Ortho Rev, 1990. 19(8): p. 681-686.
47. Donelson R, *McKenzie methods of care for mechanical low back pain: Part 1. Mechanical assessment and classification.* Revue de Medicine Orthopedique, 2000. 60: p. 4-10.
48. Donelson R, *McKenzie methods of care for mechanical low back pain: Part 2. Assessment reliability, diagnostic power, and treatment outcomes.* Revue de Medecine Orthopedique, 2000. 60: p. 11-17.
49. Donelson R, *Mechanical assessment of low back pain.* Journal of Musculoskeletal Medicine, 1998. May: p. 28-39.
50. Donelson R, et al., *A prospective study of centralization of lumbar and referred pain: A predictor of symptomatic discs and anular competence.* Spine, 1997. 22(10): p. 1115-22.
51. Donelson R, et al. *Pain response to end-range spinal motion in the frontal plane: a multi-centered, prospective trial.* in *International Society for the Study of the Lumbar Spine.* 1991. Heidelberg, Germany.
52. Donelson R, et al., *Pain response to repeated end-range sagittal spinal motion: a prospective, randomized, multi-centered trial.* Spine, 1991. 16(6S): p. 206-12.
53. Donelson R and McKenzie R, *Mechanical assessment and treatment of spinal pain,* in *The Adult Spine: Principles and Practice,* J.W. Frymoyer, Editor. 1997, Lippincott-Raven Publishers: Philadelphia. p. 1821-1835.
54. Donelson R, et al. *The low back pain experience: A natural history survey.* in *The Dartmouth/Northern New England Primary Care Cooperative Research Network annual meeting.* 2001. The Balsams, NH.
55. Donelson R, et al. *The low back pain experience: a natural history survey.* in *North American McKenzie Conference.* 2000. Orlando, FL.
56. Donelson R, Silva G, and Murphy K, *The centralization phenomenon: its usefulness in evaluating and treating referred pain.* Spine, 1990. 15(3): p. 211-13.
57. Eddy D, *Clinical decision making: from theory to practice: a collection of essays from The Journal of the American Medical Association.* 1996, Sudbury, MA: Jones and Bartlett Publishers.
58. Fennell A, Jones A, and Hukins D, *Migration of the nucleus pulposus within the intervertebral disc during flexion and extension of the spine.* Spine, 1996. 21: p. 2753-7.
59. Fordyce W, *Behavioral methods for chronic pain and illness.* 1976, St. Louis: Mosby.
60. Foster N, et al., *Management of nonspecific low back pain by physiotherapists in Britain and Ireland.* Spine, 1999. 24(13): p. 1332-42.
61. Friedman T, *The world is flat: a brief history of the twenty-first centery.* 1st ed. 2005, New York, New York: Farrer, Straus and Giroux.
62. Fritz J, et al., *An examination of the reliability of a classification algorithm for subgrouping patients with low back pain.* Spine, 2006. 31: p. 77-82.
63. Fritz J, Delitto A, and Erhard R, *Comparison of classification-based physical therapy with therapy based on clinical practice guidelines for patients with acute low back pain: a randomized clinical trial.* Spine, 2003. 28(13): p. 1363-71.
64. Fritz J, et al., *Interrater reliability of judgments of the centralization phenomenon and status change during movement testing in patients with low back pain.* Archives of Physical Medicine and Rehabilitation, 2000. 81: p. 57-61.
65. Fritz J and George S, *The use of a classification approach to identify subgroups of patients with acute low back pain: inter-rater reliability and short-term treatment outcome.* Spine, 2000. 25(1): p. 106-14.

66. Frymoyer J, *Back pain and sciatica*. New England Journal of Medicine, 1988. 318: p. 291-300.
67. Galbraith J, *The affluent society*. 1958, New York, New York: Houghton Mifflin Company.
68. George S and Delitto A, *Clinical examination variables discriminate among treatment-based classification groups: a study of construct validity in patients with acute low back pain*. Physical Therapy, 2005. 85: p. 306-14.
69. Greenhalgh T, et al., *Diffusion of innovations in service organizations: systematic review and recommendations*. The Millbank Quarterly, 2004. 82(4): p. 581-629.
70. Hertzman-Miller R, et al., *Comparing the satisfaction of low-back pain patients randomized to receive medical or chiropractic care: results from the UCLA low-back pain study*. American Journal of Public Health, 2002. 92: p. 1628-33.
71. Hestboek L and Leboeuf-Yde C, *Are chiropractic tests for the lumbo-pelvic spine reliable and valid? A systematic critical literature review*. Journal of Manipulative and Physiological Therapeutics, 2000. 23: p. 258-75.
72. Karas R, et al., *The relationship between non-organic signs and centralization of symptoms in the prediction of return to work for patients with low back pain*. Physical Therapy, 1997. 77(4): p. 354-60.
73. Kent P and Keating J, *Classification in nonspecific low back pain: what methods do primary care clinicians currently use?* Spine, 2005. 30: p. 1433-40.
74. Kent P and Keating J, *Do primary-care clinicians think that nonspecific low back pain is one condition?* Spine, 2004. 29: p. 1022-31.
75. Kilby J, Stigant M, and Roberts A, *The reliability of back pain assessment by physiotherapists, using a "McKenzie algorithm"*. Physiotherapy, 1990. 76(9): p. 579-83.
76. Kilpikoski S, et al., *Interexaminer reliability in low back pain assessment using the McKenzie method*. Spine, 2002. 27: p. E207-14.
77. Klenerman L SP, Stanley I, et al., *The prediction of chronicity in patients with an acute attack of low back pain in a general practice setting*. Spine, 1995. 20: p. 478-84.
78. Koes B, Malmivaara A, and van Tulder M, *Trend in methodological quality of randomized clinical trials in low back pain*. Best Practice & Research Clincal Rheumatology, 2005. 19: p. 529-39.
79. Koes B, et al., *Clinical guidelines for the management of low back pain in primary care. An international comparison*. Spine, 2001. 26: p. 2504-2514.
80. Kopp J, et al., *The use of lumbar extension in the evaluation and treatment of patients with acute herniated nucleus pulposus, a preliminary report*. Clinical Orthopedics, 1986. 202: p. 211-8.
81. Larsen K, Weidick F, and Leboeuf-Yde C, *Can passive prone extensions of the back prevent back problems? A randomized, controlled intervention trial of 314 military conscripts*. Spine, 2002. 27: p. 2747-52.
82. Laslett M, et al., *Centralization as a predictor of provocation discography results in chronic low back pain, and the influence of disability and distress on diagnostic power*. The Spine Journal, 2005. 5: p. 370-80.
83. Laslett M and Williams M, *The reliability of selected pain provocation tests for sacroiliac joint pathology*. Spine, 1996. 19(11): p. 1243-9.
84. Leboeuf-Yde C, Lauritsen J, and Lauritzen T, *Why has the search for causes of low back pain largely been nonconclusive?* Spine, 1997. 22(8): p. 877-81.
85. Leggett S, et al., *Restorative exercise for clinical low back pain: a prospective two-center study with 1-year follow-up*. SPINE, 1999. 24: p. 889.
86. Li L and Bombardier C, *Physical therapy management of low back pain: An exploratory survey of therapist approaches*. Physical Therapy, 2001. 81(4): p. 1018-28.
87. Loeser J, *Perspectives in pain*, in *Clinical pharmacy and therapeutics*, T. P, Editor. 1980, Macmillan: London. p. 313-6.

88. Long A, *The centralization phenomenon: its usefulness as a predictor of outcome in conservative treatment of chronic low back pain.* Spine, 1995. 20(23): p. 2513-21.

89. Long A, Donelson R, and Fung T. *Do acute and chronic and common low back pain and sciatica have more important similarities than differences?* in *International Society of the Study of the Lumbar Spine.* 2005. New York City, NY: Poster presentation.

90. Long A, Donelson R, and Fung T, *Does it matter which exercise? A randomized controlled trial of exercise for low back pain.* Spine, 2004. 29(23): p. 2593-2602.

91. Lund T, et al., *Physical work environment risk factors for long term sickness absence: prospective findings among a cohort of 5357 employees in Denmark.* British Medical Journal, 2006. doi 10.1136/bmj.38731.622975.3A.

92. Luo X, et al., *Estimates and patterns of direct health care expenditures among individuals with back pain in the United States.* Spine, 2004. 29: p. 79-86.

93. Lurie J, Birkmeyer N, and Weinstein J, *Rates of advanced spinal imaging and spine surgery.* Spine, 2003. 28: p. 616-20.

93b. Machado L, et al., *The McKenzie method for low back pain: a systematic review of the literature with a meta-analysis approach.* Spine, 2006. 31: p. E254-62.

94. Main C and Burton A, *Economic and occupational influences on pain and disability*, in *Pain management: an interdisciplinary approach*, C. Main and C. Spanwick, Editors. 2000, Churchill Livingstone: Edinburgh. p. 63-88.

95. Malmivaara A, et al., *Applicability and clinical relevance of results in randomized controlled trials: the Cochrane review on exercise therapy for low back pain as an example.* Spine, 2006. 31(13): p. 1405-9.

96. Manniche C, *Personal communication*, R. Donelson, Editor. 2003: Odensa, DK.

97. Manniche C and Gam A, *Low back pain: frequency, management, and prevention - from a Health Technology Assessment perspective.* Danish Institute for Health Technology Assessment. Vol. 1. 1999.

98. McCombe PF, et al., *Reproducibility of physical signs in low-back pain.* Spine, 1989. 14(9): p. 908-18.

99. McGuirk B and Bogduk N, *Evidence-based care for low back pain in workers eligible for compensation.* Occup Med (Lond), 2006. 56(Oct 17, 2006 Epub ahead of print).

100. McGuirk B, et al., *Safety, efficacy, and cost effectiveness of evidence-based guidelines for the management of acute low back pain in primary care.* Spine, 2001. 26: p. 2615-22.

101. McKenzie R, *The lumbar spine: mechanical diagnosis and therapy.* 1981, Waikanae, New Zealand: Spinal Publications.

102. McKenzie R, *Treat your own back.* 1997, Waikanae, New Zealand: Spinal Publications.

103. McKenzie R and May S, *Mechanical Diagnosis and Therapy.* Second ed. 2003, Waikanae, New Zealand: Spinal Publications New Zealand Ltd.

104. Merskey H and Bogduk N. *Spinal and radicular pain syndromes. In classification of chronic pain. Descriptions of chronic pain syndromes and definitions of pain terms.* in *International Association for the Study of Pain.* 1994. Seattle, WA.

105. Nachemson A, *Disc pressure measurements.* Spine, 1981. 6: p. 93-7.

106. Nachemson A, *The lumbar spine. An orthopedic challenge.* Spine, 1976. 1(1): p. 59-71.

107. NCQA, *Patient-centered physician profiling.* 2006, http://www.ncqa.org/Communications/News/SCRP_PublicComment.htm.

108. Nelson B, et al., *Can spinal surgery be prevented by aggressive strengthening exercises? A prospective study of cervical and lumbar patients.* Archives of Physical Medicine & Rehabilitation., 1999. 80: p. 20-5.

109. Oleske D, et al., *Risk factors for recurrent episodes of work-related low back disorders in an industrial population.* Spine, 2006. 31(7): p. 789-98.

110. Pedersen P, *Prognostic indicators in low back pain.* Journal of Royal College of General Practice, 1981. 31: p. 209-16.

111. Petersen T, et al., *The effect of McKenzie therapy as compared with that of intensive strengthening training for the treatment of patients with subacute or chronic low back pain: A randomized controlled trial.* Spine, 2002. 27: p. 1702-9.

112. Philadelphia P, *Philadelphia panel evidence-based clinical practice guidelines on selected rehabilitation interventions for low back pain.* Physical Therapy, 2001. 81(10): p. 1641-74.

113. Phillips H and Grant L, *The evolution of chronic back pain problems: a longitudinal study.* Behaviroal Research Therapy, 1991. 29: p. 435-41.

114. Potter N and Rothstein J, *Intertester reliability for selected clinical tests of the sacroiliac joint.* Physical Therapy, 1985. 65(11): p. 1671-5.

115. Rasmussen C, et al., *Rates of lumbar disc surgery before and after implementation of multidisciplinary nonsurgical spine clinics.* Spine, 2005. 30: p. 2469-73.

116. Razmjou H, Kramer J, and Yamada R, *Inter-tester reliability of the McKenzie evaluation of mechanical low back pain.* Journal of Orthopedic & Sports Physical Therapy, 2000. 30(7): p. 368-83.

117. Riddle D and Rothstein J, *Intertester reliability of McKenzie's classifications of the syndrome types present in patients with low-back pain.* Spine, 1994. 18(10): p. 1333-44.

118. Rogers E, *Diffusion of innovations, 4th edition.* 1995, New York, NY: The Free Press.

119. Roland M, *Point of view: the course of back pain in primary care.* Spine, 1996. 21: p. 2838.

120. Rosen C, *Association of Ethical Spine Surgeons.* 2006.

121. Schenk R, Jazefczyk C, and Kopf A, *A randomized trial comparing interventions in patients with lumbar posterior derangement.* Journal of Manipulative and Physiological Therapeutics, 2003. 11(2): p. 95-102.

122. Schnebel B, et al., *A digitizing technique for the study of movement of intradiscal dye in response to flexion and extension of the lumbar spine.* Spine, 1988. 13(3): p. 309-12.

123. Seffinger M, et al., *Reliability of spinal palpation for diagnosis of back and neck pain. A systematic review of the literature.* Spine, 2004. 29: p. E413-25.

124. Senstad O, Leboeuf-Yde C, and Borchgrevink C, *Frequency and characteristics of side effects of spinal manipulative therapy.* Spine, 1997. 22: p. 435-40.

125. Seroussi R, et al., *Internal deformations of intact and enucleated human lumbar discs subjected to compression, flexion, and extension loads.* Journal of Orthopedic Research, 1989. 7(1): p. 122-130.

126. Shah J, Hampson W, and Jason M, *The distribution of surface strain in the cadaveric lumbar spine.* Journal of Bone and Joint Surgery, 1978. 60B: p. 246-51.

127. Shekelle P, et al., *Congruence between decisions to initiate chiropractic spinal manipulation for low back pain and appropriateness criteria in North America.* Annals of Internal Medicine, 1998. 129: p. 9-17.

128. Shepherd J, *In vitro study of segmental motion in the lumbar spine.* Journal of Bone and Joint Surgery, 1995. 77B: p. S2:161.

129. Skytte L, May S, and Petersen P, *Centralization - its prognostic value in patients with referred symptoms and sciatica.* Spine, 2005. 30: p. E(293-9).

130. Smedley J, et al., *Natural history of low back pain: a longitudinal study in nurses.* Spine, 1998. 23: p. 2422-6.

131. Snook S, et al., *The reduction of chronic nonspecific low back pain through the control of early morning lumbar flexion: a randomized controlled trial.* Spine, 1998. 23: p. 2601-7.

132. Spitzer W, LeBlanc F, and Dupuis M, *Scientific approach to the assessment and management of activity-related spinal disorders (The Quebec Task Force).* Spine, 1987. 12(7S): p. S16-21.

133. Spratt K, *Statistical relevance*, in *Orthopaedic Knowledge Update: Spine 2*, e.a. D.F. Fardon, Editors, Editor. 2002, The American Academy of Orthopaedic Surgeons: Rosemont, Illinois. p. 497-505.

134. Spratt K, et al., *A new approach to the low back physical examination: behavioral assessment of mechanical signs*. Spine, 1990. 15(2): p. 96-102.

135. Spratt K, et al., *Efficacy of flexion and extension treatments incorporating braces for low-back pain patients with retrodisplacement, spondylolisthesis, or normal sagittal translation*. Spine, 1993. 18(13): p. 1839-49.

136. Sufka A, et al., *Centralization of low back pain and perceived functional outcome*. Journal of Orthopedics and Sports Physical Therapy, 1998. 27(3): p. 205-12.

137. Tauben D, *Invited Review: Central nervous system modulation of spinal pain: pain sensitization and implications for surgical selection*. SpineLine, 2005. Nov/Dec.: p. 7-12.

138. Toffler A and Toffler H, *Revolutionary wealth: shaping tomorrow's way of life*. 2006, New York, New York: Alfred A. Knopf. 512.

139. Triano J, McGregor M, and Doyne M. *Criterion-related validity of manual diagnostic maneuvers*. in *North American Spine Society annual meeting*. 1996. Vancouver, British Columbia, Canada.

140. Udermann B, et al., *Can a patient educational book change behavior and reduce pain in chronic low back pain patients?* The Spine Journal, 2004. 4: p. 425-35.

141. Ursiny J, Starz T, and al. e. *Managing the costs of care for low back pain: experience within a large health care delivery system*. in *Presented at the annual meeting of the American College of Rheumatology*. 2000. Philadelphia.

142. van den Hoogen H, et al., *The prognosis of low back pain in general practice*. Spine, 1997. 22: p. 1515-21.

143. van Tulder M, et al., *European guidelines for the management of acute non-specific low back pain in primary care*. 2004.

144. van Tulder M, et al., *Exercise therapy for low back pain*. Spine, 2000. 25(21): p. 2784-96.

145. Von Korff M, *Studying the natural history of back pain*. Spine, 1994. 19(18 Suppl): p. 2041S-2046S.

146. Von Korff M, et al., *Back pain in primary care. Outcomes at 1 year*. Spine, 1993. 18(7): p. 855-62.

147. Von Korff M and Saunders K, *The course of back pain in primary care*. Spine, 1996. 21: p. 2833-2837.

148. Waddell G, *Editorial: Subgroups within "non-specific" low back pain*. Journal of Rheumatology, 2005. 32: p. 395-6.

149. Waddell G, *A new clinical model for the treatment of low-back pain*. Spine, 1987. 12(7): p. 632-44.

150. Waddell G, McCulloch J, and Venner R, *Nonorganic physical signs in low-back pain*. Spine, 1979. 5(2): p. 117-25.

151. Waddell W, *The back pain revolution*. 1999, New York, NY: Churchill Livingstone. 438.

152. Wasiak R, Kim J, and Pransky G, *Work disability and costs caused by recurrence of low back pain: longer and more costly than in first episodes*. Spine, 2006. 31: p. 219-25.

153. Waxman R, Tennant A, and Helliwell P, *A prospective follow-up study of low back pain in the community*. Spine, 2000. 25(16): p. 2085-90.

154. Weinstein J, et al., *United States' trends and regional variations in lumbar spine surgery: 1992–2003*. Spine, 2006. 31: p. 2707–2714.

155. Wennberg J and Cooper M, *The quality of medical care in the United States: A report of the Medicare program (Dartmouth atlas of health care 1999)*. 1999, Hanover, New Hampshire: The Center for the Evaluative Clinical Sciences, Dartmouth Medical School. 167-74.

156. Werneke M and Hart D, *Categorizing patients with occupational low back pain by use of the Quebec Task Force classification system versus pain pattern classification procedures: discriminant and predictive validity.* Physical Therapy, 2004. 84: p. 243-54.
157. Werneke M and Hart DL, *Centralization phenomenon as a prognostic factor for chronic low back pain and disability.* Spine, 2001. 26(7): p. 758-65.
158. Werneke M, Hart DL, and Cook D, *A descriptive study of the centralization phenomenon. A prospective analysis.* Spine, 1999. 24(7): p. 676-83.
159. Wetzel T and Donelson R, *The role of repeated end-range/pain response assessment in the management of symptomatic lumbar discs.* The Spine Journal, 2003. 3: p. 146-54.
160. Williams M, et al., *A comparison of the effects of two sitting postures on back and referred pain.* Spine, 1991. 16(10): p. 1185-91.
161. Wilson L, et al., *Intertester reliability of a low back pain classification system.* Spine, 1999. 24(3): p. 248-54.

Index

Printed in the United States
73700LV00005BA/34